Intermittent Fasting – 2 Books in 1!

The Only Weight Loss Guide You Need to Read to Burn Fat and Keep it Off for Good. Learn How to Detoxify Your Body with the 16/8 Fasting Method!

Intermittent Fasting

Discover how to Detoxify Your Body, Burn Fat and Lose Weight with the Amazing 16/8 Fasting Method - Weight Loss Strategies to Stop Aging and Live Longer Included!

By

Nancy Johnson

© Copyright 2021 by Nancy Johnson

The following eBook is reproduced below with the goal of providing information that is as accurate and reliable as possible. Regardless, purchasing this eBook can be seen as consent to the fact that both the publisher and the author of this book are in no way experts on the topics discussed within and that any recommendations or suggestions that are made herein are for entertainment purposes only. Professionals should be consulted as needed prior to undertaking any of the action endorsed herein. This declaration is deemed fair and valid by both the American Bar Association and the Committee of Publishers Association and is legally binding throughout the United States. Furthermore, the transmission, duplication, or reproduction of any of the following work including specific information will be considered an illegal act irrespective of if it is done electronically or in print. This extends to creating a secondary or tertiary copy of the work or a recorded copy and is only allowed with the express written consent from the Publisher. All additional rights reserved. The information in the following pages is broadly considered a truthful and accurate account of facts and as such, any inattention, use, or misuse of the information in question by the reader will render any resulting actions solely under their purview. There are no scenarios in which the publisher or the original author of this work can be in any fashion deemed liable for any hardship or damages that may befall them after undertaking information described herein.

Additionally, the information in the following pages is intended only for informational purposes and should thus be thought of as universal. As befitting its nature, it is presented without assurance regarding its prolonged validity or interim quality. Trademarks that are mentioned are done without written consent and can in no way be considered an endorsement from the trademark holder.

Table of Contents

Introduction..9
Chapter 1 - How to Follow an Intermittent Fasting Protocol........11
Chapter 2 - Add more Fibers to Your Intermittent Fasting Protocol
....36
Chapter 3 - Add more Proteins to Your Intermittent Fasting Protocol..45
Chapter 4 - Add more Fruits to Your Intermittent Fasting Protocol
....53
Chapter 5 - How to Properly Integrate Vitamin B12 During an Intermittent Fasting Protocol..57
Chapter 6 - How Vitamins Can Improve Your Intermittent Fasting Protocol...64
Chapter 7 - The Detoxifying Power of Vitamin C........................71
Chapter 8 - How to Choose the Right Intermittent Fasting Protocol for You..78
Conclusion..98

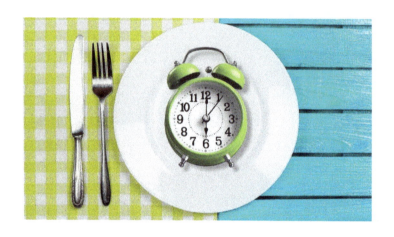

Introduction

Most women over 50 feel as if they have lost their ability to be attractive, healthy and feel good in their own bodies. But what is the cause for this widespread issue? The fact is that in today's world we are spending more and more time at home and we have significantly reduced our need for food. However, even if we do not need as many calories as we did in the past to survive and be healthy, most of us are still eating as if they were running a marathon a day.

Therefore, it should not come as a surprise that most women over 50 years of age are out of shape, overweight and unhealthy. This normally translates into a worse quality of life and is something that is frustrating for a substantial portion of the female population. Thanks to researches and scientific studies conducted by incredible nutritionists, it is now possible to overcome the negative effect of a sedentary life. In fact, intermittent fasting seems like the perfect solution for all those women that want to burn fat, lose weight and gain a healthy and new lifestyle.

The need of all these women is what inspired the writing of this guide. In fact, in the next chapters you are not going to find complicated explanations of scientific topics that, even if interesting, do not give you a clear direction on what you can do to start feeling better. On the contrary, while writing this book, a great effort was made to make sure that each concept is followed by a subsequent strategy that can be implemented in a healthy intermittent fasting protocol.

By reading this book you will get all the information and practical steps you need to follow to start intermittent fasting in just a few days. We advise you to talk to your doctor before changing your diet as intermittent fasting is not suitable if you have certain healthy conditions.

Please, be aware that the goal of this book is to give you accurate information on intermittent fasting, but it does not take the place of a true medical advice. We hope that you can find motivational and informative insights that help you make a change for the better.

Chapter 1 - How to Follow an Intermittent Fasting Protocol

As we have seen in previous chapters, it can be very frustrating to feel overweight, without considering the associated health risks. You can lose self-confidence and even become a little lazy. To adequately improve health conditions, it is necessary to change diet and choose healthier dishes, controlling the portions. When starting an intermittent fasting protocol, make sure you are getting enough nutrients and avoid restricting your food intake too much. A diet is most effective when accompanied by a healthy lifestyle and the right attitude.

Ask yourself why you want to follow an intermittent fasting protocol

By having all the reasons and goals of your diet clear, you can choose a sensible meal plan that pays off all your efforts. These are only a few of the different reasons why you might want to start an intermittent fasting protocol.

- Manage diabetes. If you are diagnosed with this disease, you need to change your eating habits. The key to living well with such a disorder is to cut back on sugars or cut them out of your diet.
- Reduce the risk of heart disease. By eating foods that lower cholesterol and help you shed excess abdominal fat, you can decrease the likelihood of heart disease.
- Get rid of the pounds accumulated during pregnancy. It is normal to gain weight when pregnant, but once you have given birth, you can decide to regain your silhouette.
- Get ready for summer. Many women go on a diet at the beginning of summer, when they are terrified of wearing a bathing suit. Sometimes small changes in eating style are enough to avoid this fear and not to be caught unprepared for the costume test.

Before starting any intermittent fasting protocol, you should consult your doctor to be sure that it does not adversely affect your health condition. Tell him that you intend to follow an intermittent fasting protocol. Any meal plan below 1200 calories per day can be dangerous. Michelle May, a weight management specialist, argues that "rapid weight loss from drastically reducing calories results in the loss of fluids, fat and muscle mass. Therefore, metabolism slows down and the body needs fewer calories to survive". In addition, the body tends to accumulate a greater amount of body fat, with the risk of developing metabolic syndrome and type 2 diabetes.

Some women use calories to calculate how much food they should eat, others base their intermittent fasting protocol in grams (of proteins, carbohydrates, etc.), others draw up a list of dishes to eat more often and those to eat less often. Decide how you intend to manage your intermittent fasting protocol.

Make sure your intermittent fasting protocol is compatible with the medications you take. You must be sure that your meal plan complies with nutritional guidelines and that it has no contraindications in relation to the drug therapies you are following.

For example, if you are treating hypertension with the ACE inhibitors used, you need to keep your consumption of bananas, oranges and green leafy vegetables under control. If you have been prescribed tetracyclines, you will probably need to avoid dairy products while taking these drugs.

Analyze your current eating habits

Before starting, you need to be aware of your daily diet. So, try to write down what, when and where you eat to get to know your current eating habits.

Put a diary it in the kitchen or near the bed and write down what you consume (dishes, snacks, small "tastings" from other people's dishes, without leaving anything out), the time and place where you eat (in the kitchen, on the sofa, in bed).

Everyone has their own eating habits and "triggers" that lead them to overeat. Awareness is the first step in learning how to properly manage these aspects when adopting a new meal plan. These are some of the most common triggers for women of your age.

- One of the biggest causes of overeating is stress. When we feel out of sorts or anxious, we often try to console ourselves with food. In these cases, you may want to adopt some stress management techniques or stock up on healthier foods to keep this trigger under control.
- It is more difficult to make correct food choices when we are tired. If you have a tendency to gorge on food when you feel powerless, you probably want to rest

and go to the grocery store once you regain your energy.
- If you have a tendency to empty the refrigerator when you are alone, you may want to consider adding some activity or hobby to your meal plan that will keep you busy outside the home and prevent you from eating compulsively.
- If you skip meals when you have a busy day, you'll arrive hungry at dinner time and eat whatever comes your way. In these circumstances, think about including moments in your new diet when you have the opportunity to eat something in your teeth.

Most dieters find it appropriate to count calories, but another overwhelming majority say they don't actually know their calorie needs. We are used to thinking that fewer calories means losing weight more easily, but in reality it is necessary to be aware of the food sources they come from, not just the quantities to be consumed.

Women report that they consume an average of 1800 calories per day. If you are trying to lose weight, your requirements are likely to be even lower, but you should never go below 1200 calories per day, otherwise the body thinks that it is in a state of starvation, and it begins to store fat.

Ask a dietician or personal trainer to help you figure out how many calories you should be taking in daily to lose the extra pounds in a healthy way. Consider how much physical activity you do during the day. Prioritize foods rich in fiber (whole grains) and protein (lean meats). They will help you feel full for longer and provide you with more energy. Avoid "empty" calories that don't give your body the right fuel. Alcohol and foods such as potato chips are great examples of low-nutrient calorie sources.

Follow the guidelines for healthy eating

The Ministry of Health has developed guidelines in the food sector to help the population to eat properly and follow a balanced diet. In other words, you have the ability to know what the right portions are for each food group without indulging in some of them. In addition, you also need to vary your diet by ranging between different food groups, not just eating apples or other types of fruit, for example. Additional important recommendations include: reducing daily calories from added sugars by 10%; decrease daily calories from saturated fat by 10%; consume less than 2,300 mg of sodium per day. Additionally, there are specific instructions regarding the amount of foods you should try to consume each day, including the following ones.

- Eat nine servings of fruit and vegetables a day. A portion of fruit is equivalent to about 150 grams, which is a medium-sized fruit or 2-3 small ones. As for vegetables, one serving corresponds to 250 grams of raw vegetables or 50 grams of salad.

- Eat six servings of grains a day and make sure half of them are whole grains. One serving of cereal is equivalent to a slice of bread or 80 grams of rice or pasta.

- Eat two or three servings of dairy products a day, but try to choose low-fat ones. 240ml of milk equals one serving.

- Eat two or three servings of protein a day. One serving corresponds to 100 grams of meat, or the size of a palm, an egg, 16 grams of peanut butter, 28 grams of nuts and 50 grams of beans.

- Try the "rainbow diet", which is a diet that varies from the point of view of colors (blueberries, red apples, asparagus, etc.). Each color corresponds to different nutrients and vitamins.

Consume more lean protein

The body needs to strengthen muscles, support immunity and keep metabolism fast. To benefit from protein intake without experiencing the disadvantage of consuming fat, opt for leaner sources. Choose skim milk instead of whole milk and lean ground beef or turkey instead of very marbled cuts. Check for hidden fat in meat dishes.

Avoid whole milk derivatives, offal such as liver, fatty and highly marbled meats, ribs, cold cuts, hot dogs dressed with sauces, bacon, fried or breaded meat and egg yolk.

Let yourself be conquered by the fish. Certain types of fish are rich in omega-3 fatty acids, which are substances that can lower the triglyceride index in the blood. You can increase your omega-3 intake by choosing cold-water fish species, such as salmon, mackerel and herring.

Don't underestimate the beans. Also consider peas and lentils. Generally, legumes are excellent protein sources that do not contain cholesterol and have less fat than meat. Try a soy or bean burger, or add some diced tofu to stir-fried veggies or salad.

Consume whole foods

Whole grains are whole grains made up of three parts: germ, bran and endosperm. Therefore, whole foods contain all three components. Unfortunately, carbohydrate foods undergo a refining process that eliminates the bran and germ, resulting in a loss of about 25% of protein and at least 17 key nutrients. To get all the benefits, opt for foods that are labeled in full on the package.

According to some studies, a diet rich in whole grains has numerous benefits, including reducing the risk of heart attacks, heart disease, type 2 diabetes, inflammation, colorectal cancer, gum infections and asthma. They also help maintain a healthy weight, improve carotid artery health and blood pressure. So, don't hesitate to include about 48 grams of whole grains in your daily diet.

Look for them when you shop. 15-20% of food products on supermarket shelves consist of whole grains. So, look for those that carry the "wholemeal" label or look for a product that is made from whole grains or flours.

Diversify the consumption of carbohydrates. There are not only flour and bread, but also pasta, cereals, biscuits, wraps, scones and other products based on wholemeal flour, so read the packaging carefully.

Include healthy fats

Not all fats are bad for your health. In fact, some should definitely be included in your meal plan. Monounsaturated fatty acids (MUFA) and polyunsaturated fatty acids are appropriate because they provide some benefits, such as lowering bad cholesterol (LDL) and increasing good cholesterol (HDL), but they also help stabilize insulin and blood sugar levels.

Foods high in monounsaturated fatty acids include avocado, canola oil, nuts (almonds, cashews, pecans and macadamias, nut butter), olive oil, olives, and peanut oil.

Eliminate trans fats. They are contained in hydrogenated vegetable oils, so you can spot them if you find "hydrogenated oil" written on the labels. They increase bad cholesterol and lower good cholesterol, with the consequent risk of heart disease, cancer, heart attacks and infertility.

Major sources of trans fat include industrially fried and prepackaged foods, especially baked ones.

Beware of products that pretend to be free of trans fat. For example, in the United States, the Food and Drugs Administration (FDA) authorizes "trans fat free" if a particular food contains up to half a gram per serving. Imagine, then, that if consumption is high, every half gram can become an excessive amount. As far as the European Union is concerned, a regulation has not yet been established that regulates the content of trans fats in food products or the related labeling within the Member States. Trans fats are so bad for your health that New York City has passed a law banning their use in restaurants.

Read the labels

By paying attention to the nutritional tables on the packaging, you can stick to a healthy choice of your foods. One very important part of the table is the portion information: it suggests how many portions are contained in each pack and what the nutritional data are for each of them.

It's convenient, fast and easy to eat out or buy ready-made meals. However, you cannot control the preparation of the food or the ingredients used. One of the most effective ways to lose weight is to cook at home. You can choose healthier cooking methods (such as baking instead of frying) and fresh ingredients.

By drawing up a weekly menu, you will be less likely to let the situation get out of hand and order takeaways in the middle of the week. You can make your life easier by preparing healthy dishes to freeze and consume according to your needs.

Try to enjoy cooking. Give yourself a new set of knives or a cute apron. This way, you will find the right motivation to spend more time in the kitchen.

Don't neglect snacks. Good news! You can indulge in a snack while following your intermittent fasting protocol. By eating more snacks, you can speed up your metabolism and help your body burn more calories throughout the day. In fact, a healthy snack also helps reduce hunger and keep you from overeating at mealtimes.

The secret lies in the choice of food. Consume fresh fruits and vegetables, nuts or low-fat dairy products. Try a few slices of cucumber with chickpea hummus for a satisfying afternoon snack.

Keep healthy snacks on hand when you are at work. If you have some toasted almonds in your desk drawer, you will be less likely to go looking for cookies left behind by a colleague on a break.

Season your dishes

If they are appetizing, you won't be able to resist the temptation to eat them. To add flavor to dishes and stay healthy, try dressing them with some sauce. For example, you could pour tomato puree instead of butter over baked potatoes to lower your fat and calorie intake. Moreover, it is also a way to enrich the meal with other vegetables.

If you season chicken, fish and salads with some sauce, you can make your dishes more varied and interesting. Try buying a fresh salsa at the supermarket or make your own.

You can flavor almost any dish by adding spices and herbs. By the way, they are all calorie-free. Try buying parsley, rosemary, or thyme. They will make your chicken, pork or salad recipes more succulent and original.

In addition to the flavor, some ingredients are also good for your health. For example, garlic has anti-inflammatory properties. Use it to season fish or soups - you'll get a healthy and appetizing meal. Turmeric is another fairly used spice that should never be missing in the pantry. Try adding it to salad dressings to add flavor.

Avoid popular intermittent fasting protocol

It can be very tempting to try the latest trend in intermittent fasting protocols. Often, newspapers and television networks report the experiences of famous women who have successfully tried the most popular slimming treatments. However, it is important to remember that not only are they ineffective, they can also have adverse health effects.

Most popular intermittent fasting protocols focus on one food group, such as carbohydrates. On the contrary, a healthy diet involves the intake of different foods, which is a program that includes the intake of all nutrients. Avoid diets that require you to eliminate the consumption of certain categories of foods.

Some crash diets can harm the body, because they promote a very low calorie intake, causing serious health dangers. Rather, get the recommended amount of calories for your build and make healthy choices.

Avoid industrially produced foods. Processed foods and ready meals are rich in substances that should be avoided like sodium, saturated fats and sugars. This does not mean that a fast food hamburger or frozen food will kill you, but they are foods that you should limit.

The Dietary Guidelines for Americans recommend not consuming more than 10% of calories from saturated fat. If you follow a daily diet of 1500 calories, it means that you can eat 15 grams of saturated fat per day. Fast-food burgers contain between 12 and 16 grams.

Stay away from sugary drinks. Sugary drinks, especially soft drinks, promote weight gain and obesity. The calories that we take safely from the straw are always calories and contribute to accumulating pounds, so try to remove or reduce their consumption.

The most thirst-quenching drink is and always has been water. Also, by consuming more of it, you will feel fuller and can decrease the amount of food you consume during meals. You can improve its taste by adding a few slices of lemon, cucumber, mint or other fresh ingredients.

Fruit juice looks healthy, especially if it is 100% pure, but it contains a lot of sugar. Drink it in moderation or add a little water for beneficial nutritional effects with fewer calories. In a study conducted by researchers at Harvard University, the consumption of sugary drinks is linked to 180,000 deaths worldwide per year, including 25,000 in the United States alone. Another study dating back to 2013, conducted by scientists at Imperial College London, found that the risk of type 2 diabetes increases by 22% for every 340g of sweetened drinks consumed daily.

Avoid certain ingredients depending on your health condition

If you have a digestive disorder that prohibits you from taking certain ingredients, read labels carefully and stock up on products that fit your dietary needs. Follow these guidelines and ask your doctor for medical advice before starting an intermittent fasting protocol.

- Celiac disease. Celiac disease is a chronic inflammation of the small intestine caused by intolerance to gluten, a protein found in wheat, rye and barley. Thanks to a greater awareness of the needs of gluten intolerant subjects, it is possible to find various gluten-free products not only in specialized shops, but also in normal supermarkets.

- Hypertension. It is a dangerous disease that precedes heart disease and heart attack. It can be partly managed with a diet rich in fruits, vegetables and lean proteins. The DASH diet - acronym for "Dietary Approaches to Stop Hypertension", or nutritional approach to reduce hypertension - has been shown to lower blood pressure. It is recommended by various health organizations, including the U.S. National Institutes of Health, and has been ranked the best diet of 2012 by the U.S. News and World Report, a US communications company that publishes news, opinion, consumer advice and market analysis.

- Food allergy. If you suspect you have a food allergy, get allergy tests. Eight foods are responsible for 90% of all food allergies: peanuts, nuts, milk, eggs, cereals, soy, fish and shellfish. If you are allergic, read the packaging carefully to avoid products that can trigger allergic reactions.

While you may be tempted to cut your calorie needs drastically and set high expectations to accelerate weight loss, a slow, determined approach will be more effective and easier to maintain.

Change only one meal a day. Instead of suddenly starting an intermittent fasting protocol, try to introduce only one healthier or smaller meal per day. By gradually changing your diet, you will not feel deprived of anything, but you will have time to adjust to the new situation.

Move your body

A proper intermittent fasting protocol allows you to start adopting a healthier lifestyle. However, you will see better results if you also start exercising. According to some studies, combining diet and physical activity results in health benefits and weight loss.

Try to exercise at least an hour a day. You can break it down into steps of a few minutes to make it more manageable. For example, try walking to work and climbing stairs instead of driving and taking the elevator.

Get some rest

If you don't get enough sleep, you are more likely to gain weight. When you can't rest, your body produces more cortisol, the stress hormone, causing you to seek comfort in food rather than encouraging you to make healthier choices.

Try to sleep for 7-9 hours every night. This way, you will tend to have a healthier body weight than when you only sleep 5-6 hours. Avoid using devices that emit blue light (smartphones, tablets, laptops, and televisions) at least half an hour before bed, as they can keep you awake. Try to keep the pace. If you go to bed at the same time every night and wake up at the same time every morning, you will be more active and rested.

Check your progress

To keep track of your improvements, establish a system that allows you to see how you are doing. The food diary you started writing to keep track of old eating habits can be a great tool to know which way you are headed. Compare your progress, temptations, and successes each week.

Enter all the information relating to your new food plan (starting weight, target weight, daily menus) in a software that monitors your evolution. Many programs also offer healthy recipes and provide forums where you can connect with other people who share your goals.

Check your weight every week. It is not only the daily diet that matters, but also what the scales say. Establish a day a week to weigh yourself and write down the results you have achieved.

Set goals that will allow you to improve your health. To have a healthy lifestyle, you need to learn to set realistic goals. Don't make impossible claims, like "lose 7 lbs in a month". Instead, set smaller, more achievable goals. Typically, to lose weight properly, you need to lose 1lbs per week. Set yourself manageable goals, such as working out six days a week. This way, you will be able to accomplish them more easily and you can reward yourself every time you reach a small milestone. Avoid food-based rewards; give yourself a new tracksuit or a pair of sneakers.

Pay attention to food. Nowadays it is very common to eat while watching TV, checking your cell phone or about to go out, but there is a risk of gulping down more than you need. When it's time for lunch or dinner, eliminate all distractions and sit down at the table. Focus on the food in front of you and appreciate its scent, appearance, taste and texture. Put your fork down between bites to give yourself time to chew thoroughly.

Stop once you've reached your goal

Some intermittent fasting protocols are real lifestyles that can be followed continuously, while others are designed to achieve specific goals in a shorter period of time. Many are fine if they last for a while, but in the long run they risk not being healthy.

Pay attention to the "yo-yo" effect. Also known as weight cyclicality, it is the phenomenon in which the cyclical loss and regain of body weight occurs following various diets. It can cause psychological distress, dissatisfaction and binge eating and, over time, damage the cells that line blood vessels, increasing the risk of heart disease.

Ending an intermittent fasting protocol can be a relief, but if you resume your old eating habits, you risk regaining the weight you lost so hard. Instead, try a maintenance program to stay fit.

If you have followed an intermittent fasting protocol based on liquid foods or which has significantly limited calorie intake, you must be careful to gradually reintroduce solid foods into your diet so as not to traumatize the body. Consume homemade soups, fruits and vegetables for a few days before adjusting to a healthy eating routine.

Stay positive and get a healthy picture of your body.

The strength of positive thinking is not a chimera. In fact, it is crucial to eat a balanced diet. It can keep motivation high, but also energy. On the other hand, negative thoughts can promote bad behavior, such as hitting on food to satisfy emotional hunger and skipping workouts.

Don't be negative. Try not to blame yourself if you go wrong and eat pizza instead of something healthier. Instead, get back on track the next day.

Some days it is difficult to feel comfortable in your own skin. It mostly happens if you are constantly surrounded by extraordinarily thin figures of famous people. However, it is very important for general health and well-being to have a positive body image: it increases your self-esteem and predisposes you to make healthy choices.

Focus on the best aspects of your body. If you love your arms, say it when you look in the mirror. Get in the habit of complimenting yourself at least once a day.

Record a thought-provoking sentence or quote when you mirror yourself. By encouraging yourself every day, over time you will be able to develop a more positive body image.

Be kind to yourself

According to some research, if you are more forgiving of yourself, you will be able to get back into shape more easily. When a negative thought comes to you, try to recognize it and then let it go. It really doesn't make sense to blame yourself for missing a session at the gym. It is much more effective to forgive yourself and move on.

Tell someone (or everyone) that you are following an intermittent fasting protocol. By declaring it, you will prepare yourself to successfully carry out your business, because you will take responsibility in front of others. You may also count on the support of family and friends who will encourage you to achieve your goal.

Stick encouraging phrases on the refrigerator. By having wise words that can lift your mood, you will be able to face the most difficult days of your diet.

Don't deprive yourself of everything that makes you feel good. Go to a beauty center, go to the hairdresser, buy a new perfume. Anything that makes you feel special and pampered can make up for the lack that sometimes creeps in when following an intermittent fasting protocol.

We are sure that if you follow these tips you are going to feel amazing while following your intermittent fasting protocol.

At this point you should have all the basic information you need to get started. In the next chapters we are going to dive deeper into specific topics concerning intermittent fasting.

Chapter 2 - Add more Fibers to Your Intermittent Fasting Protocol

The importance of dietary fiber is considerable. Dietary fiber, in fact, has a series of beneficial effects, such that it is an integral part of any balanced diet in the name of health.

Before discussing in detail the functions of dietary fiber and the reasons why it is important, it is necessary to review what exactly dietary fiber is.

What dietary fibers are

In nutrition, it is called dietary fiber, or simply fiber, all that set of organic substances belonging to the category of carbohydrates (with rare exceptions), which the human digestive system, with its digestive enzymes, is unable to digest. and absorb.

Dietary fibers are found mainly in foods that have a plant origin, such as fruit, vegetables, whole grains and legumes.

Depending on whether or not it is soluble in aqueous solution, dietary fiber is distinguished, respectively, in: soluble dietary fiber and insoluble dietary fiber.

Soluble fibers

When it is inside the intestinal lumen, soluble dietary fiber becomes, by virtue of its solubility, a viscous gelatinous substance, with chelating properties against macronutrients such as carbohydrates and lipids. Being viscous, soluble fiber slows intestinal transit, causing a sense of fullness.

The main sources of soluble fiber are: legumes, oats, barley, fresh fruit, broccoli and psyllium seeds.

Insoluble fibers

When found in the intestine, insoluble dietary fiber absorbs water, which has the effect of increasing the volume of stool and making it softer. Thanks to the consequences described above, dietary fiber speeds up intestinal transit, interfering with the absorption of nutrients and reducing the time spent in the intestine of toxic substances for the intestinal mucosa.

The main sources of insoluble fiber are: whole grains, green leafy vegetables, courgettes, flax seeds and dried fruit.

Properties and benefits of dietary fibers

Today, with increasing insistence, experts in the wellness sector, such as dieticians, nutritionists, doctors and personal trainers, are keen to emphasize the leading role that dietary fiber plays in a healthy diet.

In fact, dietary fibers have the following benefits.

- They regularize intestinal function, opposing disorders such as constipation, hemorrhoids and diverticulitis;

- They interfere with the absorption of lipids (fatty acids and cholesterol) and carbohydrates (i.e. sugars), making it a very valuable ally in the fight against obesity and diseases caused by failure to control blood sugar, cholesterol and/or triglyceridemia, such as diabetes mellitus, coronary heart disease, atherosclerosis, high cholesterol and hypertriglyceridemia;

- By speeding up intestinal transit, they reduce the time spent in the intestine of toxic substances for the intestinal mucosa, which has a protective effect against colon and rectal cancer;

- They favor the maintenance of an intestinal pH that depresses the growth of that harmful intestinal bacterial flora, whose activity is a source of metabolites known to be associated with the development of colon and rectal tumors; parallel to this, they stimulate the growth of that beneficial intestinal bacterial flora (prebiotic effect), with protective effects on the intestinal mucosa;

- By causing a feeling of fullness, they increase the sense of satiety, which contributes to better control of body weight and the fight against overweight and obesity.

Importance of soluble dietary fibers: the benefits

Soluble fiber is the type of dietary fiber that is the protagonist of the fight against obesity and diseases caused by the lack of control of glycemia, cholesterolemia and triglyceridemia; therefore, the protective action against excess weight and diseases such as diabetes mellitus, coronary heart disease, atherosclerosis, hypercholesterolemia and hypertriglyceridemia depends on the soluble fiber.

Furthermore, soluble fiber is responsible for that improvement in intestinal pH that depresses the growth of harmful bacteria residing in the intestine, whose activity is associated with colon and rectal cancers, and, at the same time, enhances the development of beneficial bacteria, through a prebiotic effect.

Importance of insoluble dietary fiber: the benefits

Insoluble fiber is the type of dietary fiber protagonist of the opposition to disorders characterized by slow intestinal transit (therefore constipation, hemorrhoids and diverticulitis) and to neoplasms that arise from the excessive permanence of toxic substances in the intestine (i.e. colon and rectum).

Are you getting enough fiber while following an intermittent fasting protocol? Probably not. Do you think that to do this it is necessary to eat only salads? Not at all! Read this chapter to know how to consume fibers while following an intermittent fasting protocol.

Find out how much fiber you need

We have already mentioned the importance of keeping a diary dedicated to what you eat each day, including the amount of food you consume. Research each food on the internet and note the fiber it contains. Here are how many fibers you need depending on your age.

- Men under 50: 38 grams of fiber per day.
- Men over 50: 30 grams of fiber per day.
- Women under 50: 25 grams of fiber per day.
- Women over 50: 21 grams of fiber per day.

If you are currently introducing 10 grams per day, don't jump to 21 the next day. You need to give the natural bacteria in the digestive system time to adjust to your new ingestion. The changes should therefore take place within a few weeks.

Start with breakfast

If it's high in fiber, you can probably add 5-10 grams more to your daily diet.

Eat grains with 5 or more grams of fiber per serving. If you can't stop eating your favorite grains, add a few tablespoons of unprocessed wheat bran or mix them with high-fiber grains. If you like toast in the morning, make it with wholemeal or high-fiber bread. Cook muffins containing whole grains or unprocessed wheat bran.

Add fruits such as berries, raisins, or bananas to the grains to increase fiber intake by 1-2 grams. Swap refined white flour for oat or flax flour if you're making pancakes, and you'll add 1-2 grams of fiber per serving.

If you're making pancakes and waffles, use 2/3 of all-purpose flour and 1/3 of wheat bran. Swap quick-cook oats for traditional oats for an additional 2-4 grams of fiber per serving.

Eat the peel of fruits

Incorporating more fruits and vegetables into your diet will bring more fibers in, but only if you eat the peel as well. For example, don't peel apples or potatoes (in the latter case, use the peels to make snacks). You also need to know that by leaving the peel on the potatoes when cooking them, you will get more vitamins and minerals from the pulp. Do not eat the green parts of the peel, they do not taste very good.

Here are a few interesting meal ideas to increase the fiber intake.

- Dry pea soup, a nutrient-dense food: one cup contains 16.3 grams of protein.
- Vegan roast made with nuts and dried peas.
- Sunflower seed cream and dried peas.
- Iraqi shorbat rumman pomegranate soup.
- Dry pea burgers.
- Spinach and dried peas.

Add whole grains or unprocessed wheat bran to stews, salads, vegetables, and baked foods (meatloaf, bread, muffins, cakes, and cookies). You can also use ground flaxseed or coconut flour, two other great sources of fiber.

Eat more whole grains, which are higher in fiber because the husk was not removed during the preparation process. In addition to providing you with more fiber, they will help you lose weight. A diet rich in whole grains changes your body's response to glucose and insulin, which accelerates the breakdown of fat and makes it easier to dispose of subcutaneous fat, which you can see and grasp.

Replace white bread with wholemeal bread. If you can't, make sandwiches using one slice of white bread and one slice of wholemeal bread. Do you prepare it at home? Replace white flour with whole or half whole wheat flour (use a little more yeast or let the dough rise longer and add an extra teaspoon of baking powder for every 2 cups of whole wheat flour).

Eat wholemeal pasta. If you don't like the taste of it, mix it with the refined one or season it more, but don't overdo it. Eat more brown rice or add barley to white rice for more fiber. You will barely taste the barley, especially if you season rice. Eat more beans, which are high in fiber and protein (which are used to build muscle mass).

Just by following these simple tips you will make sure that you get all the fibers you need to keep your body healthy and in shape.

Chapter 3 - Add more Proteins to Your Intermittent Fasting Protocol

As we have seen at the beginning of the book, protein is an essential nutrient for the development and cell growth of the human body, and is important for supporting the body's immune system. Also, adding protein to your intermittent fasting protocol can improve your health and your overall metabolism, especially if you want to lose weight. The amount of protein you should be getting daily varies based on your gender and health goals. To add protein to your diet, you must first determine the ideal amount of protein to consume each day, and then incorporate foods that are higher in protein into your diet. Use this chapter as a guide to determine the daily amount of protein you need, and find out how you can add it to your diet.

Consult your doctor for the ideal daily protein intake. Your doctor can check the correct dose of protein you should be taking each day based on your health status and the goals you want to achieve.

Eat the right amount of protein each day based on your gender. According to the "Dietary Reference Intake" (DRI) system used by health professionals in the United States and Canada, women over 50 should consume 46 gr. of protein per day.

If your goal is to lose weight, increase your daily protein intake. If you intend to add more protein to your diet specifically in order to lose weight, know that you can take up to 120g. of protein per day; however, this dose may vary based on your gender and health status. Replace the meat included in your diet with lean meats. Examples of lean meats that are high in protein are chicken, turkey, fish, or fillet of meat.

Add cottage cheese to your diet. Each 1 cup (236.58 ml) of fresh cottage cheese contains approximately 28 g. of protein. Add fruit or almonds to cottage cheese to enhance the flavor.

Add eggs to your diet. You can choose whether to eat only egg whites or whole eggs; the yolk contains about 6.5 gr. of protein.

Throughout the day, snack on nuts, grains, and seeds. Sunflower seeds, chickpeas, edamame beans, unsalted peanuts, and peanut butter are all examples of high-protein foods.

Add yogurt to your diet. Yogurt is generally a high-protein food, especially Greek yogurt, as it is often denser and richer in protein than regular yogurt.

Eat high-protein vegetables. Examples of particularly high-protein vegetables are broccoli, spinach, cauliflower, asparagus, mushrooms, onions and potatoes.

Eat raw vegetables (such as salad), or cook the vegetables by frying or steaming them. These preparation methods will allow the vegetables to keep all the nutrients and proteins intact; boiling vegetables can reduce the amount of nutrients found in them.

If necessary, use protein powders or protein supplements. Protein powders can be added to certain foods or beverages to increase your daily protein intake, especially if you are having trouble meeting your daily protein intake through the foods you already consume.

Add vanilla-flavored protein powder to your coffee, or mix the powder into foods you cook to enhance the flavor, such as pancakes, oatmeal or muffins.

Since there are many different protein powders out there, in the next few pages we are going to tell you how to choose the best brand for your needs.

Protein powder

One way to integrate protein into your diet is through the use of protein powders. The market is full of protein powders, so it's important to know the differences between the products and choose the one that's right for you.

Before adding protein powders to your intermittent fasting protocol, you should know why you want to do it. This way you can choose the protein or combination of proteins that will give you the desired effect.

Add protein powder to build muscle. They are a great way to help with muscle regeneration and building new muscles. If you are training to gain muscle mass, it is a good idea to add them to your diet. However, a supplement should never replace true food sources of protein. It's all about that, supplements. You will need to use them to add extra protein to your diet that cannot be taken with food.Add protein powder to lose weight. Protein increases the feeling of satiety and fullness, limiting your desire to eat. They are also important for maintaining current muscle mass when exercising.

Add protein powders for your overall health. Studies have shown that some proteins help transport bioactives around the body and lower cholesterol. Adding protein powders to a healthy intermittent fasting protocol can help reduce cholesterol, blood pressure, or fat mass faster than a healthy diet without them.

Add protein powder as a dietary supplement. There are many reasons for adding protein powder as a dietary supplement.
- Vegetarians often do not get adequate amounts of protein and need supplements.
- People who have gastric bypass need extra protein due to reduced nutrient absorption.
- People with certain diseases or disorders, such as celiac disease or Crohn's disease, may need extra protein during breakouts due to reduced absorption by the gut.

Protein is stored in the muscles of the body and must be consumed daily or it will be absorbed by the muscles for biological tissue repair. The result would be the reduction of muscle mass and the loss of strength. For this reason, it is recommended that women take the essential amino acids required by the body every day. Most women living in the Western world don't need extra protein because their intermittent fasting protocol is high in protein. This does not mean that using protein powder is bad for your health, but that you will need to plan your diet carefully, including protein powders as a source of nutrition. Research is still ongoing to determine the exact number of proteins for each of us to consume. However, there are recommendations, based on scientific evidence, that everyone can follow.

Get 15% of your daily calories with protein. Each gram of protein contains 4 calories. So in the case of a 2000 calorie diet, you should eat 75g of protein per day. Again, these are values suitable for sedentary people and the minimum quantities necessary to sustain life. Active people are expected to double that percentage, to 30%.

Increase your daily calorie intake from protein by up to 40% (with fats at 30% and carbohydrates at 30%). Extra protein should replace refined carbohydrates (avoid high fructose corn syrup and processed grains). For a healthy adult, this increase shouldn't adversely affect your kidneys if you drink

12 glasses of water a day. By increasing the calories you ingest with protein, you will receive the heart-beneficial effects brought by these nutrients, burn fat and gain lean mass.

Limit your protein intake to 0.8 - 1.25g per 0.5kg of weight per day if you are looking to gain muscle mass and decrease fat mass. If you have any health problems that can affect your kidneys, limit protein to 0.8 per 0.5kg of weight and consult your doctor for frequent blood tests to check your kidney function. The American Diabetes Association makes this recommendation for people with kidney disease or diabetes. Take note of the proteins you ingest with a food diary.

Chapter 4 - Add more Fruits to Your Intermittent Fasting Protocol

Eating healthily is a very important part of a healthy intermittent fasting protocol. Fruit is essential to our intermittent fasting protocol because it contains many vitamins, minerals, carbohydrates and fiber. Here are some easy-to-follow tips for getting more fruit into your intermittent fasting protocol and improving your overall well-being.

Eating fruit on a daily basis can help you maintain a healthy weight and reduce the risk of heart disease, stroke, and some forms of cancer. In addition, fruit contains a large variety of vitamins, minerals, carbohydrates and fiber. Hence, eating the right fruit combinations brings significant benefits. For example, an apple contains a lot of fiber but little vitamin C; But if you add an orange and a few strawberries, you'll get all the vitamin C you need for the day.

Eat five servings of fruit a day if your intermittent fasting protocol allows for it

Many countries have adopted national or regional programs to encourage people to eat at least five servings of fruit and vegetables a day. One glass of fruit juice counts as one serving, but drinking five will always count as one serving. If a third of your diet consists of fruits and vegetables, you are well on your way to a healthy diet.

Adding sliced banana to cereal or dehydrated fruit to oatmeal, or making a fresh fruit salad are all great ways to liven up your breakfast. A handful of blueberries and raspberries can be of great benefit. In fact, in addition to the usual benefits offered by fruit, they also contain antioxidants that protect against DNA damage. These include slowing down the skin aging process and preventing sun damage to the skin; a good start to any day.

Use fruit to snack on

Fruit is the perfect food to consume on the go, and can easily replace cookies, cakes and chocolate when snacking. High-fat, high-sugar snacks contain few essential vitamins and minerals, as well as low fiber, and can lead to poor digestion. So, keep some fruit in your car, purse or on your desk at work, to overcome those energy drops that hit you in the mid-morning or mid-afternoon.

Most food manufacturers enthusiastically insist on the fruit content in their food, to make you think it is a great food. Be careful, though. In fact, not everything that has the word "fruit" in its name is what it seems. Remember to check the fat and sugar content in frozen fruit desserts. Canned fruit in fruit juice is usually fine, but beware of canned fruit in syrup, which may be full of sugar. Try to eat five servings of fruit a day for a week. You will see how good it makes you feel.

Eat your favorite fruit within 20 minutes of waking up. During sleep, your body fasts for nearly eight hours. Eating fruit within 20 minutes of waking up rehydrates your body and provides it with low-glycemic carbohydrates that keep your metabolism going throughout the day.

Chapter 5 - How to Properly Integrate Vitamin B12 During an Intermittent Fasting Protocol

Vitamin B12, also known as cobalamin, is one of the water-soluble B vitamins. Others include folic acid, biotin, niacin, thiamin, riboflavin, vitamin B5 (pantothenic acid), and vitamin B6. All B vitamins play a fundamental role in the production of energy and for this purpose B12 plays an even more important role, which also extends to the production of red blood cells and the proper functioning of the metabolism and the central nervous system. In the next few pages we are going to tell you how to supplement vitamin B12 during an intermittent fasting protocol.

Eat quality seafood

One of the best ways to integrate B12 into your intermittent fasting protocol is to eat seafood. For example, lobster, shellfish and especially clams contain a high amount of vitamin B12. Fish, such as trout, salmon, tuna, and haddock, are also excellent sources of B12. An 85g serving of seafood contains nearly 400% of the daily cobalamin requirement, while an 85g serving of clams far exceeds the daily allowance.

Both meat and offal of beef, such as liver, contain a lot of B12 as well. Pork is also an excellent source of this vitamin. On average, one slice of beef liver contains 2800% of the recommended daily requirement of vitamin B12. Some meat replacement foods such as tofu are fortified with vitamin B12. Consider this option if you are vegetarian or vegan and check the product label for the amount of B12 it contains.
White meats also provide B12, as do eggs. Two cooked eggs contribute greatly to the daily cobalamin requirement.

Do not forget dairy products

To increase your B12 intake, include dairy products such as yogurt, milk and cheese in your intermittent fasting protocol.

Some types of plant-based milk are also fortified with this vitamin.

A snack of 250g of low-fat fruit yogurt gives you half your daily B12 requirement.

Try whole grains

Many breakfast cereals are high in vitamin B12. By combining fortified cereals, eggs and milk at the first meal of the day, you will be able to take the recommended daily dose of cobalamin from the moment you wake up.

For example, a bowl (just over 40g) of low-fat muesli with raisins contains 10mcg of vitamin B12, which is 417% of the recommended daily allowance.

Whole grains are a great way for vegans and vegetarians to get B12, since plant-based foods don't contain high levels of this vitamin.

Yeast products and nutritional yeast are excellent sources of vitamin B12. To increase your intake, you can add nutritional yeast to any dish, from cereals to smoothies to evening meals. 5 g of nutritional yeast fortified with vitamin B12 contains more than twice the daily dose of this vitamin.

Take a vitamin B12-only supplement

You can also buy a vitamin B12 supplement in pills. Cobalamin is best absorbed along with other vitamins. Therefore, take it with B6, magnesium, niacin, or riboflavin. In order to get a B12 supplement, you can ask your doctor for a prescription. They may advise you to take this vitamin in the form of an injection or gel.

The recommended daily dose to stay healthy is 2.4 mcg for women over the age of 50. Pregnant and breastfeeding women should take 2.8 mcg.

It is also essential for children, but their needs may be lower than the aforementioned values. The amount needed varies according to age: 9 to 13 years equals 1.8 mcg, 4 to 8 years 1.2 mcg, 1 to 3 years 0.9 mcg, 7 to 12 months 0.5 mcg and from 0 to 6 months at 0.4 mcg.

If you are vegan or vegetarian you should keep the level of this vitamin under strict control. Some women who follow a vegetarian or vegan intermittent fasting protocol may experience a deficiency of vitamin B12, because one of the main sources of vitamin B12 is made up of foods of animal origin. Cobalamin can be obtained through the consumption of fortified cereals. Try eating 3-4 servings a day of B12-enriched foods.

Symptoms of vitamin B12 deficiency

A cobalamin deficiency leads to exhaustion, weakness, diarrhea, constipation, decreased appetite and weight loss. There are also other symptoms produced by B12 deficiency on the nervous system, which include numbness and tingling in the hands and feet, balance problems, confusion, depression, behavioral changes, irritation of the mouth or tongue, and bleeding of the gums. The likelihood of B12 deficiency increases with age, so be careful if you are a woman over 50.

This problem affects women who suffer from atrophic gastritis, pernicious anemia, Crohn's disease, celiac disease, or immune system disorders, such as Graves' disease or lupus. It also occurs in women undergoing partial surgical removal of the stomach and small intestine and in people who drink a lot. Prolonged use of heartburn medications can also cause a vitamin B12 deficiency.

Before taking a vitamin B12 supplement you should talk to your doctor, especially if you are on drug therapy. Taking cobalamin does not involve risks. In fact, in the medical literature there are no toxic or side effects reported. However it could interact with some classes of drugs used in the treatment of gastroesophageal reflux and peptic ulcer. The drugs used to treat these conditions decrease the absorption of vitamin B12. Furthermore, some drugs used to treat diabetes and cholesterol can also reduce its absorption.

If you are taking any of these medications, ask your doctor if you need to increase your B12 intake.

If you have any symptoms of vitamin B12 deficiency, you should see your doctor for a diagnosis. Symptoms of insufficient cobalamin intake can be related to various ailments that need to be diagnosed by your doctor.

If you have been diagnosed with vitamin B12 deficiency, visit your doctor regularly and follow their advice regarding a correct vitamin B12 supplementation.

If you follow these instructions, you will have no issues during your intermittent fasting protocol, even if you are a vegan or vegetarian.

Chapter 6 - How Vitamins Can Improve Your Intermittent Fasting Protocol

Vitamins and minerals perform several important tasks for the body and are essential for maintaining good health while following an intermittent fasting protocol. Most of the need for these elements is met with food and a balanced diet. In addition to helping you take the recommended daily amount, vitamin and mineral supplements also help you lose weight, but you still need to follow an appropriate and balanced diet plan, as well as exercise regularly.

Ask a doctor for professional advice

Before taking any over-the-counter drugs (or supplements), you must speak to a doctor. In fact, food supplements are not always safe for all people.

Although vitamin, mineral and herbal supplements are subjected to careful checks by the Ministry of Health, they are commercially available without a prescription and anyone can buy any kind. Therefore, it is important to receive the right advice and warnings from the doctor, before starting to take any type of supplement, to avoid unpleasant side effects.

Contact your doctor when you think you want to start vitamin treatment so that you know which one is most appropriate for you. Tell them about the goal you want to achieve with this treatment and ask them if there are other possible solutions besides taking vitamins.

If you want to ask your doctor about the supplements you have already purchased, remember to tell them the brand, the type of vitamin and the format (these are on the package label), as well as the appropriate dosage. This information helps your doctor determine if it is a suitable product for your specific needs.

Read the label

Since there are countless products on the market (not always of certain origin), you need to be aware of what you ingest when taking supplements. Check carefully what you decide to take.

Read the directions for all vitamins. For example, if you are looking for a vitamin D supplement, choose a product that clearly says "vitamin D", then read the label to know all the ingredients, so you know the format and all the ingredients. other excipients present. Make sure other substances are also safe for you.

Check the size of the tablet and the dosage of the active ingredient. Nutritional values should also be included in the label. The recommended posology (for example, 2 tablets) and the amount of active substance contained in each dose (for example, 30 mg) should be indicated. Make sure you know precisely the appropriate dosage for your needs and the correct amount of active ingredients contained in the tablets. Do not take more than the recommended daily amount.

Like prescription drugs, many over-the-counter supplements can also have contraindications. Check for any adverse effects on the label and search online for more information if needed.

Take vitamin D supplements

Studies have shown that people who regularly take this dietary supplement (and were previously deficient in it) while following an intermittent fasting protocol lose more weight than those who do not.

Vitamin D deficiency is a major nutritional deficiency, affecting approximately 500 million women worldwide. The side effects of the deficiency of this important substance are many and include: increased mortality, cancer, metabolic disorders, diseases of the skeletal system, heart problems and infections.

Currently, the recommended daily dosage is 400 IU. However, more recent studies recommend taking up to 2000 IU per day if you are following an intermittent fasting protocol.

Vitamin D is fat-soluble, which means that it accumulates in the adipose layer of the body and can remain in the body for up to 3-6 months. You have to be careful not to take too much, as if it is present in the body in excessive quantities, it becomes toxic and can no longer be eliminated from the body.

Vitamin D is present in few and rare food sources. However, you can find it in the following foods: cod liver oil, fortified milk and orange juice, salmon, beef liver, eggs and swordfish.

Take calcium supplements

Some studies have found that calcium, combined with vitamin D, helps you lose weight. In fact, it has been found that taking large amounts of calcium discourages the accumulation of fat in the cells; in addition, it can bind to some fats in foods, preventing the body from absorbing them.

The recommended daily dosage is 1000-1200 mg. However, you should divide this amount into 500 mg doses, as the body cannot absorb more at a time.

Recent research has found that higher calcium levels can cause heart disease and harden arteries. Pay attention to the total amount you take in through the supplements and foods you eat.

The best food sources are dairy products, dark leafy vegetables, broccoli and almonds.

Take magnesium

It is an important mineral that stimulates over 300 chemical reactions in the body. Studies have shown that, in addition to these functions, it also promotes weight loss.

Magnesium plays an important role in many metabolic functions, but it has been found to improve fasting glucose and insulin levels, thereby helping to regulate weight. A deficiency in this mineral can lead to irritability, muscle weakness and arrhythmia. The recommended daily dosage is 350 mg. Take one or two tablets throughout the day. The best food sources are dairy products, beans, nuts, fish and seafood.

The role of probiotics

Although not considered vitamins or minerals, these are supplements that have been shown to be effective in losing fat and maintaining optimal weight.
Probiotics are "good" bacteria that are alive and present in various points of the gastrointestinal tract. They are ingested through food and drink; their purpose is to strengthen the immune system, as well as prevent or manage constipation and diarrhea.

Several studies have found that consuming various types of "good" bacteria and enriching the intestinal flora are two aspects associated with weight loss and maintaining a "healthier" weight.

If you want to include these supplements in your diet, get ones that contain at least 5 billion CFU (colony forming units) per serving.

You can also eat foods that are rich in it, such as yogurt with active cultures or yogurt to drink, sauerkraut, miso, and tempeh.

Choline supplements

Studies have shown that it helps reduce weight and overall body mass. Choline does not fall into the category of vitamins or minerals, but it is an essential nutrient that acts on metabolism, lipid transport and hormone synthesis.

The recommended daily dosage for a woman over 50 following an intermittent fasting protocol is around 400-500 mg. However, specific choline supplements usually contain about 13% of the active ingredient, but generic ones that contain 3500-4000 mg of phosphatidylcholine (the lead group contains choline) are just as safe.

Among the best food sources of choline are beef liver, eggs, wheat germ, scallops and salmon.

Chapter 7 - The Detoxifying Power of Vitamin C

Vitamin C is one of the most important vitamins for the body; you can get it through your diet by eating foods such as oranges, red peppers, cabbage, broccoli and strawberries. You can also take it in large quantities through powdered supplements to mix with water (or other drinks), as it is believed to be able to relieve ailments such as stress, various diseases and hormonal imbalances. Before you cleanse yourself with this method, however, you need to take precautions and talk to your doctor to evaluate the risks and potential benefits. An abundant intake of vitamin C is not safe for anyone and caution should be taken. However, if you have chosen this option, set up and complete the process within two to three hours; if you experience any complications during cleansing, contact your doctor immediately.

Talk to your doctor if you have irritable bowel syndrome (IBS) or hemochromatosis. If you have IBS or an iron deficiency such as hemochromatosis, you must seek the advice of the doctor before deciding to take a large amount of vitamin C because, if you proceed on your own, these diseases can worsen in the presence of high amounts of acid. ascorbic; your doctor can recommend a specific dosage taking into account your health condition. [1]

You should also avoid this vitamin if you have kidney disease or are concerned that you are allergic to ascorbic acid.

Do not take more than 3000 mg per day. Higher dosages can cause blood clots, kidney stones, digestive problems and other heart-related ailments; you don't have to risk overdosing by taking too much at once. [2]

Doses greater than 2000 mg per day can cause cramps, chest pain, dizziness, diarrhea, fatigue, heartburn and intestinal problems; if you are concerned about these symptoms, consult your doctor before taking vitamin C.

If you are pregnant or breastfeeding, you must be especially careful in consuming this vitamin, as in high doses it can cause hypertension; you must always speak to the gynecologist to find out if it is safe for you, for the baby and not to proceed if you do not have his consent.

Tell your doctor if you have vomiting or diarrhea when you cleanse with vitamin C. If you feel really sick, vomit or have diarrhea when starting treatment, you may be allergic or intolerant to the active ingredient stop taking it immediately and contact your doctor right away. [3]

If you experience a feeling of general discomfort or lightheadedness that does not go away after an hour of starting the process, stop and see your doctor.

Look for buffered vitamin C. Pure powder can be aggressive to the stomach and cause ailments such as heartburn and inflammation. Preferably look for the buffered form, which also contains minerals such as calcium, magnesium and zinc and which is gentler on the digestive system. [4]

You can get it online or in health food stores.

Take powdered ascorbic acid. It is an alternative and contains sodium bicarbonate in addition to the vitamin; this extra ingredient regulates the water intake and facilitates the digestion of vitamin C. [5]

You can look for it online and in health food stores.

Have plenty of filtered or purified water available. You need it to dissolve the vitamin C powder; you have to drink a lot of it during purification to help the substance travel throughout the body and stimulate defecation. [6]

You must drink at least 5 or 6 glasses of water during the procedure, after which you can drink as many to recover from detox.

Organize yourself not to carry out any demanding activities during the treatment. The whole procedure can generally last from two to six hours, depending on the time it takes for the vitamin to travel throughout the body. Do not schedule outings during this time, as you will need to have easy access to the bathroom to expel the water and vitamin C powder.

Start the treatment immediately in the morning. Proceed as soon as you get up and before breakfast; in this way, the body can absorb the precious vitamin. [8]

Take 1000 mg of vitamin C dissolved in water every hour. Add this dose of vitamin C powder (in buffered form or ascorbic acid) to half a glass of drinking water, mix with a spoon and sip. [9]
If you don't like the flavor of the vitamin powder, you can add some fruit juice with no added sweeteners.

Repeat the treatment until you start producing watery stools. Continue drinking 1000 mg of powdered vitamin C dissolved in half a glass of water every hour; proceed for an hour or two or until you feel the need to go to the bathroom. Check for watery stools this is a sign that you are cleansing your body with this substance. [10]

It takes a few hours for the intestines to start emptying; be patient; you may need to go to the bathroom within 2-4 hours of starting treatment.

Note the times you take the vitamin during the process. Make sure you keep track of the frequency and hourly dosage; that way, you know your vitamin intake for sure and make sure you don't overdo it. [11]

Also take note of when you make liquid stools to better understand how much vitamin you need to detoxify the body, especially if you plan to repeat the treatment in the future.

Consume liquid meals during the procedure. Cleansing leads to better results if you don't eat large amounts of solid foods; opt for fluid foods, such as soups or broths, so as not to create an upset stomach. Continue like this for the 2-4 hours of treatment and gradually return to solid foods when finished. [12]

Drink plenty of water during your cleanse to help the vitamin pass through the digestive tract.

Insert solid foods like rice, quinoa, and cooked vegetables after the "cleanup" is done. After a couple of days, you can switch to more consistency proteins like fish, tofu, beef, and chicken.

Gradually reduce your vitamin intake. Once your body is cleansed, take a smaller dose of the substance daily for 4-5 days; continue in this way until you reach less than 1000 mg / day. [13]

This gradual decrease guarantees the adaptation of the organism to this change and prevents the purification from having negative effects on the intestine.

You may still notice some water in the stool during this phase, but the situation should normalize when you reach a dosage of 1000mg.

Repeat the cleanse every four months or when you start feeling unhealthy. If you have a chronic flu or cold symptoms, follow the treatment every four months or so, sticking to the first-time dosages for best results. [14]

You can also take 50-100 mg of vitamin C regularly to stay healthy; take it first thing in the morning, even before breakfast.

Chapter 8 - How to Choose the Right Intermittent Fasting Protocol for You

As we have seen, there is a big difference between an intermittent fasting protocol and a diet. In fact, an intermittent fasting protocol is an eating strategy that can be implemented to maximize the weight loss effects of a given diet. However, nowadays there are a lot of different diets and it could be difficult for the average woman to choose the best one for her. In this chapter we are going to examine the most common diets out there to identify which one is the best one for you to implement using an intermittent fasting protocol.

There are dozens of diets in the world, from those that are really smart and in most cases effective, to those that seem to have been invented from scratch and that are useless. In this chapter we will analyze 12 of the most popular diets, ranging from the most restrictive slimming treatments (in terms of calories and food groups), to nutritional styles based on a certain scheme (in which it is necessary to change the times and the way of eating), up to crash diets (useful when you need to quickly lose a lot of pounds). In fact, by having all the necessary information, you can choose the diet that best suits your needs and your intermittent fasting protocol.

Low-calorie diet

It is among the easiest to follow. All you need to do is decrease your calorie intake. In fact, the less you eat, the sooner you lose weight. The assumption behind this eating style is that fewer calories help you lose weight. That said, be careful not to drop below 1200 calories per day.

Advantages. you can eat whatever you want, the important thing is to control the portions. All food packages sold at the supermarket are equipped with a nutritional table. Also, in many restaurants you can find low calorie dishes. In short, it is not difficult to follow it and to integrate it into an intermittent fasting protocol.

Disadvantages. It requires some calculation and some effort, because you will have to keep track of everything you eat and drink, although it should be remembered that technology makes it easier for you. Also, if it is very restrictive, consider that you will not feel full; you may also complain of nausea and dizziness. As if that weren't enough, you'll have a hard time maintaining your weight once you start eating normally again.

Who should follow this diet? If you are determined and have no problem carrying pen and paper with you (or use an app every time you put something under your teeth), this is the diet for you. It is ideal for those women who do not have a large budget and are full of commitments. It is not recommended for those who tend to snack on a lot and for people who hate to constantly monitor everything they eat and drink.

Low-carb diet

It is able to accelerate weight loss, but it is not suitable for everyone. If you follow it, you need to prioritize the consumption of protein and fat (those who support it say that fat is good), so you will eat a lot of meat, cheese, eggs, vegetables, nuts and nothing else. The assumption behind this type of diet is that, when the body has no carbohydrates to burn, it enters a state of ketosis which leads it to directly consume fats (which is why taking them is very important).

Advantages. It is quite easy to follow and allows you to eat many tasty, often fatty foods (such as meat, cheese, etc.), which are prohibited in other diets. There is no calorie restriction, so if it's done right you will rarely feel the pangs of hunger.

Disadvantages. During the initial period (two weeks), people who follow it often feel bad. However, this is a physiological response which passes quickly. Afterwards you feel full of energy, you see an improvement in health and you lose weight. Furthermore, it may be difficult to comply with it because many foods are prohibited. Finally, it can get monotonous, especially if you're not very creative in the kitchen.

Who should follow it? If you know how to cook or are an expert in grilling, you will have no difficulty. It is also ideal for those who do not get bored of always eating the same dishes. However, it is not very suitable for those who love sweets and are not a lover of meat.

The South Beach diet

This diet is similar to the Atkins diet, in fact it eliminates the consumption of saturated fats and certain carbohydrates.

Due to its characteristics it is slightly different and some find it more manageable (because the introduction of some carbohydrates is allowed, especially in the second phase).

However, if you are on a low-carb diet, you should take at least 20g per day.

Low-fat diet

In this case, you don't have to eliminate calories and carbohydrates, but fat. It is an eating style that involves some health risks because it excludes essential fatty acids, which are important for the proper functioning of the body. The only fats that are bad for you are trans fats. In short, this diet helps you lose weight because it allows you to take in more calories, proteins and carbohydrates, while restricting the intake of fats.

Advantages. It is quite easy to follow and favors the consumption of fruit and vegetables. Also, in the supermarket you can find numerous low-fat products and avoid those that are notoriously fatty, such as sweets, cakes, cheese, red meat, etc.

Disadvantages. The main disadvantage of this diet is that a low-fat food can contain sugars and salt, substances that are equally harmful to the body, if not even less healthy. Certain lipids are good for your health and there is a risk that the body will want more carbohydrates to fill the gap left by the fat deficit.

Who should follow it? Try it if you like fruits, vegetables, whole grains and lean meats. Discard it if you are a lover of red meats and cheeses, want a meal plan that doesn't involve complications, or are looking for a quick way to lose weight.

Vegan and vegetarian diet

The vegetarian diet prohibits the consumption of meat, while the vegan diet involves the elimination of any product of animal origin (eggs, milk, etc.). That said, there are numerous variations of these two food choices. In fact, there are the flexitarians, who occasionally indulge in meat; the pescetarians, who only include the consumption of fish among their meats; ovo-vegetarians, who admit indirect animal products such as eggs. In general, they are all low-calorie, low-fat, and nutrient-rich diets.

Benefits. This type of diet allows you to lower cholesterol and blood pressure. Most vegetarians and vegans eat a lot of fruits and vegetables, which are ideal for staying healthy. It is not necessary to count calories and sweets are not prohibited. Furthermore, from an ethical point of view they are two diets respectful of animal life.

Disadvantages. You have to be careful. The organism needs proteins that vegetables often do not offer. Being vegan doesn't mean being healthy. Plus, it doesn't necessarily mean you will lose weight (in fact, a vegetarian could technically eat a whole tray of sweets).

Who should follow these diets? Try them if you don't like meat, if you are a good cook (you will have to modify the recipes to meet your dietary needs) and you don't have a tight budget (fresh products can be expensive). Avoid them if you've always been a meat lover and don't want to have complications when cooking or going out to eat.

Glycemic index diet

It is a system that is attentive to foods that can raise blood sugar levels. The higher the potential of a food to raise blood sugar (on a scale of 1 to 100), the less it is considered healthy. A diet like this makes you avoid anything that raises blood sugars, because it is assumed that the glycemic spikes lead to increased fat accumulation, an increase in appetite and weight gain. This diet involves the consumption of complex and whole carbohydrates, as well as some types of fruit and vegetables.

Benefits. It can reduce the risk of diabetes and heart attack. In addition, it favors the consumption of foods that are part of each food group. You can eat as much as you want and when you like as long as the glycemic index is low.

Disadvantages. It is an illogical diet. For example, some types of fruit are fine, while others are not (as if that weren't enough, a ripe banana has a higher glycemic index than an unripe one). As a result, it can be a bit difficult to follow. Also, as the body's reactions to food change from day to day, it can be difficult to monitor its effectiveness.

Who should follow it? Opt for this diet if you are looking for a diet that allows you to lose weight slowly and progressively. Discard it if you want fast results and an easy-to-control diet.

Mediterranean diet

It focuses on the consumption of simple and fresh foods. It is based on the typical diet of Southern Italy and Greece, consisting of numerous varieties of fruit and vegetables, olive oil, non-GMO dairy products, dried fruit and little red meat. Those living in these regions have a lower risk of developing cardiovascular disease, cancer, diabetes and obesity.

Benefits. It does not openly rule out a particular food group, although it leaves little room for industrially processed junk foods. It includes complex carbohydrates, such as oats (great for most people), and occasionally a glass of red wine. It has been shown to be good for overall health and is fairly easy to follow, as long as the follower is aware of the decision made.

Disadvantages. Weight loss is not fast and the effects may be more internal than external. Since it is quite a varied diet, it is easy to assume that a food is fine, when it could be harmful. A handful of nuts is healthy, but a whole jar is not. Sometimes it is difficult to know when to contain portions.

Who should follow it? Try it if you intend to improve your overall health (rather than lose weight quickly) and you like the idea of avoiding processed foods, preferring fresh ones while following an intermittent fasting protocol. Forget if you want a quick loss of weight, don't know how to cook (few frozen foods are compatible with this diet) or have a limited budget.

Paleo diet

It is a recently developed diet that allows you to eat only the foods available in the time of primitive men, namely lean meats, fish, fruit, non-starchy vegetables, nuts and eggs. It totally excludes dairy products, processed foods and starchy vegetables, such as potatoes. It can significantly lower your blood sugar and, therefore, prove to be very healthy.

Benefits. It can promote strong weight loss, as long as it is followed correctly. It is based on the assumption of how humans should eat to get better. Also, don't count calories!

Disadvantages. You cannot eat potatoes and dairy products, because they are included in the list of prohibited foods even if they are generally considered healthy (like milk). Moreover, since some basic ingredients are excluded, it can be really difficult to eat out or have a particular dish prepared. In addition, there is the risk of overdoing it with some dish that is good for you, provided it is consumed in moderation.

Who should follow it? Choose this diet if you are an advocate of healthy eating and like to challenge yourself in the kitchen. Avoid it if you don't have the time and energy to try new cooking techniques or don't want to make a thousand changes to the restaurant menu. Also, it's not ideal for someone who can't live without dessert.

Asian diet

Known as the mother of all modern diets, the traditional Asian diet has a history of nearly 5,000 years and is now practiced by billions of people around the world. It focused on a natural, healthy and balanced diet based on fruit, vegetables and whole grains, with moderate consumption of eggs, lean meat and fish. Those who follow it are also exposed to a lower risk of diabetes, high cholesterol, heart disease and stroke.

Benefits. It is completely natural, based on scientific research and 100% safe. It is balanced to meet all of your nutritional needs. No calculation is needed, but you can do it if you wish.

Disadvantages. You have to learn how to cook some Asian dishes, even if they are generally not complex. You have to give up almost all processed and junk foods.

Who should follow it? It is the perfect diet for those who want to eat healthily and cleanly, learn about other cultures and try new recipes in the kitchen.

Diet plans for weight loss

There is a plethora of diet programs, such as Weight Watchers, Jenny Craig and Nutrisystem, planned with menus, meetings and brochures to help you stay on track and motivated. Typically, they prescribe a low-calorie diet, but some also include low-fat foods.

Advantages. They are tailor-made for you. Some even provide for home delivery of what you need to eat. If you follow them carefully, it will be almost impossible to overshoot. In addition, you can count on a network of people ready to support you.

Disadvantages. In general, you only eat the foods included in the program, which by the way is paid for by the membership.

Who should follow it? Give it a try if you want to have something planned to help keep your life uncomplicated. It is also ideal for those women who need constant stimulation and find meetings and participation in support groups useful. However, if you like to cook and give space to creativity, this is not for you.

Cyclic diet

Recent studies are in favor of this type of diet which is divided as follows. Some days of the week are dedicated to the consumption of low-calorie foods, a couple of days are dedicated to a regular diet and only one to a high-calorie diet. This alternation prevents the body from getting used to the intermittent fasting protocol and therefore the metabolism remains active.

Advantages. There is no exclusion or limitation to any food group and there is a day in which you can "binge in a healthy way". You are not told when you can do it - you just have to organize yourself properly.

Disadvantages. You have to learn how to count calories, which can be a hassle especially in the beginning. You can't even give yourself too much freedom: just because you have a full calorie day, doesn't mean you can eat 30 cookies, otherwise you compromise the results.

Who should follow it? According to most of the research it appears that, when done correctly, it is quite healthy. If you want to see results, just make sure you consume lots of fruits, vegetables, lean meats and whole grains every day, regardless of the day. If you are a committed person and are interested in understanding how the body works, it could be for you. However, you also need to know your weaknesses. In fact, it's easy to give in to temptation, count calories and avoid losing sight of the ultimate goal.

The three-hour diet

You can eat every 3 hours to keep the metabolism active, otherwise the body will automatically run out of reserves. Eat light meals at regular times by adding a few 100-calorie snacks. However, you must avoid eating 3 hours before bedtime. If you want, you can consume precooked foods. As you can see, this goes against a standard intermittent fasting protocol as you can eat every three hours. We thought to include this diet in this list because it could be a viable option for some of you.

Benefits. You can eat everything, including less healthy dishes, as long as you can control the portions. It also helps you feel full because you eat all day and promotes a good balance between the various food groups.

Disadvantages. It could be easily mistaken. Freedom can lead you to go astray. Furthermore, there is not much scientific evidence to support the effectiveness of mini-meals.

Who should follow it? Try this diet if you feel like trying something different and are in the habit of snacking on a lot. Discard it if you want an effective method to help you lose weight fast or you don't have enough willpower to keep your commitment.

The new Beverly Hills diet
It is based on a very specific idea. In fact, for this diet it doesn't matter what you eat, but what counts is to do it at the

right time and make the right food combinations. A correct combination of these two factors promotes digestion which prohibits the body to store fat. Supporters of this dietary regimen believe it is possible to lose 7 lbsin the initial phase which lasts 35 days.

Benefits. Believe it or not, there are no restrictions on calories or food groups. You don't have to calculate your calorie intake, but pay attention to when you eat. In addition to this, the consumption of fruits and vegetables is encouraged, which is good for the body.

Disadvantages. To begin with, there is no scientific evidence to support its effectiveness; in the beginning you can only eat fruit, which is not healthy at all. The rules are a bit confusing and difficult to follow (for example, once you have chosen a protein dish, you can only eat proteins; when you eat a certain type of fruit, then you have to move on to another and so on).

Who should follow it? Try this diet if you don't get along with portion control or food restrictions. If you're willing to splurge, you can buy books, DVDs, and meal plans. Avoid it if you are not committed and diligent.

Avoid crash diets

Crash diets are extreme diets that promise rapid weight loss, but the problem is that they rarely work. They often cause you to starve and, as a result, are bad for your health. When you want to lose weight, try to avoid the following types of diets.

- Purifying diets;
- Juice diets;
- Soup-based diets, such as cabbage or chicken
- Liquid based diets;
- The grapefruit diet.

Regardless of what kind of diet you decide to adopt, co-opt someone else's support if you can. This is especially important if you have chosen a difficult diet to follow. Knowing that you can count on someone is what you need to not lose heart.

This is why programs like Weight Watchers are enjoying some success. However, you don't need to subscribe to a certain program if you want support. In fact, you can just contact friends and family to have some form of support.

Combine diet and exercise

Each diet should be paired with physical activity, whether it's aerobics, weight lifting, or both. Whether you want to walk or run 3 miles, try to get moving. This way, the results will be really visible and it will be easier to continue the diet. Do at least 150 minutes of exercise a week to keep yourself healthy. If you want to lose weight, you should increase the training time to at least 5 hours.
Avoid motor activity only if you crack down on calorie restriction. Exercising continuously on an empty stomach carries health risks.

Whether you are on a diet or not, preferably choose organic and whole foods. The less they are processed, the more the nutrients they contain are preserved. This eating style can be expensive. To save money, buy in bulk or, if you can, shop at a fruit and vegetable store. Also, if you are lucky enough to have friends who are attentive to their nutrition, try to get organized with them to buy larger quantities at a better price.

Make sure your diet is flexible and enjoyable

You will not be able to follow it if it does not have these two characteristics:

- **Flexible**. There will be days when you want to go to a restaurant, days when you have nothing at home but pizza and days when you have no desire to respect your intermittent fasting protocol. A flexible diet that doesn't cause you to feel guilty when you go wrong is easier to implement in an intermittent fasting protocol.

- **Pleasant**. You don't have to be a scientist to understand that it's not the best to drink just water with a squeeze of lemon and maple juice for a week. If it were, it would be a recommended diet for everyone. Whatever type of diet you choose, make sure it allows you to eat foods you enjoy. Do you like meat? Try the Atkins diet. Do you love olive oil? Give the Mediterranean diet a try. The choices are not lacking and your intermittent fasting protocol can be adapted to different diets.

Ask your doctor for advice

The only person who knows your body almost as much as you do and who can give you a reliable opinion is your doctor. Therefore, you need to consult it before you seriously go on a diet. Every woman is different and some diets are not suitable for everyone.

This recommendation is especially true if you are pregnant, experiencing menopause, an elderly person, or if you have health problems. The last thing to hope for is that a new eating style will affect your health in a negative way. So, select a couple of diets that piqued your interest and talk to your doctor about them before implementing them in your intermittent fasting protocol.

Ask your doctor if they can recommend a dietician who will help you make a nutritional plan that fits your lifestyle and weight loss goal.

Conclusion

We would like to thank you for making it to the end of this intermittent fasting guide. We have done our best to ensure that every information contained is useful and helps you in your journey towards a healthier you.

We know how frustrating it could be to start an intermittent fasting protocol and feeling discouraged by the fact that results do not appear immediately. As we repeated throughout this entire guide, the goal of intermittent fasting is to create a healthy lifestyle that can support you over the years, not just give you a rapid weight loss that is unsustainable over the long run.

By following the intermittent fasting protocols and strategies shared in this book, you will certainly burn fat, lose weight and feel much better. However, as we do not know you in person, our final recommendation can only be the following one.

Before starting an intermittent fasting protocol talk to your doctor and find out whether intermittent fasting could be a good idea for you or not. Remember, never sacrifice your health to fit into that new skirt you just got.

Be healthy and your weight will adapt.

To your success!

Nancy Johnson

Intermittent Fasting for Women

The Complete Guide to Lose Weight, Slow Aging, Burn Fat, Live Longer and Balance Hormones - Detoxify Your Body with the 16/8 Fasting Method!

By

Nancy Johnson

© Copyright 2021 by Nancy Johnson

The following eBook is reproduced below with the goal of providing information that is as accurate and reliable as possible. Regardless, purchasing this eBook can be seen as consent to the fact that both the publisher and the author of this book are in no way experts on the topics discussed within and that any recommendations or suggestions that are made herein are for entertainment purposes only. Professionals should be consulted as needed prior to undertaking any of the action endorsed herein. This declaration is deemed fair and valid by both the American Bar Association and the Committee of Publishers Association and is legally binding throughout the United States. Furthermore, the transmission, duplication, or reproduction of any of the following work including specific information will be considered an illegal act irrespective of if it is done electronically or in print. This extends to creating a secondary or tertiary copy of the work or a recorded copy and is only allowed with the express written consent from the Publisher. All additional rights reserved. The information in the following pages is broadly considered a truthful and accurate account of facts and as such, any inattention, use, or misuse of the information in question by the reader will render any resulting actions solely under their purview. There are no scenarios in which the publisher or the original author of this work can be in any fashion deemed liable for any hardship or damages that may befall them after undertaking information described herein.

Additionally, the information in the following pages is intended only for informational purposes and should thus be thought of as universal. As befitting its nature, it is presented without assurance regarding its prolonged validity or interim quality. Trademarks that are mentioned are done without written consent and can in no way be considered an endorsement from the trademark holder.

Table of Contents

Table of Contents..105
Introduction..108
Chapter 1 - An Introduction to Fasting.......................................110
Chapter 2 - The Basics of Nutrition..117
Chapter 3 - Benefits of Intermittent Fasting...............................138
Chapter 4 - Therapeutic Fasting...144
Chapter 5 - Training while Fasting...154
Chapter 6 - Intermittent Fasting and Aerobic Training...............159
Chapter 7 - Intermittent Fasting and Strength Training..............170
Chapter 8 - Practical Steps to Get Started with Intermittent Fasting
....178
Chapter 9 - Before Fasting..187
Chapter 10 - After Fasting..191
Conclusion..201

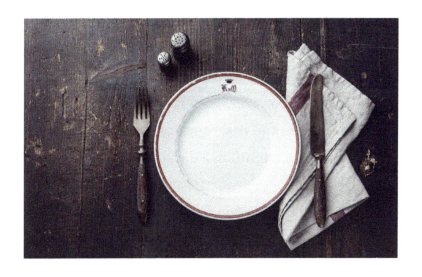

Introduction

Most women over 50 feel as if they have lost their ability to be attractive, healthy and feel good in their own bodies. This is due to the fact that in today's world, we are spending more and more time at home and we have significantly reduced our need for food. However, even if we do not need as many calories as we did in the past, most of us are still eating as if they were running a marathon a day.

Therefore, it should not come as a surprise that most women over 50 are out of shape, overweight and unhealthy. Thanks to researches and scientific studies conducted by incredible nutritionists, it is now possible to overcome the negative effect of a sedentary life. In fact, intermittent fasting seems like the perfect solution for all those women that want to burn fat, lose weight and gain a healthy and new lifestyle.

The need of all these women is what inspired the writing of this book. In fact, in the next chapters you are not going to find complicated explanations of scientific topics that, even if interesting, do not give you a clear direction on what you can do to start feeling better. On the contrary, while writing this book, a great effort was made to make sure that each concept is followed by a subsequent strategy that can be implemented in a healthy intermittent fasting protocol.

By reading this book you will get all the information and practical steps you need to follow to start intermittent fasting in just a few days. We advise you to talk to your doctor before changing your diet as intermittent fasting is not suitable if you have certain healthy conditions.

Please, be aware that the goal of this book is to give you accurate information on intermittent fasting, but it does not take the place of a professional opinion. We hope that you can find motivational and informative insights that help you make a change for the better.

To your success!

Nancy Johnson

Chapter 1 - An Introduction to Fasting

Before beginning our discussion about intermittent fasting, it is important to have a good understanding of what fasting actually is in a more general sense. In the next few pages we are going to lay out the basics for the rest of the book, so pay close to attention.

Although cases of prolonged fasting due to lack of food are extremely rare in our society, voluntary food deprivation is often undertaken for political, social or religious reasons. Since humans can survive absolute fasting for about 24-30 days, the body's physiological response to this deprivation can be divided into 4 phases, respectively called the post-absorption period, short fasting, medium fasting and prolonged fasting. Let's take a look at them one by one to understand them better.

Post-absorption period
It occurs a few hours after the last food intake, as soon as the foods introduced in the last meal have been completely absorbed by the intestine. On average it lasts three or four

hours, followed, under normal conditions, by an ingestion of food that breaks the temporary state of fasting.

In the post-absorption period there is a progressive accentuation of hepatic glycogenolysis ("breakdown" of glycogen into the individual glucose units that make it up), which is necessary to cope with the glycemic drop and supply extrahepatic tissues with glucose.

Short-term fasting

In the first 24 hours of food deprivation, metabolism is supported by the oxidation of triglycerides and glucose deposited in the liver in the form of glycogen. Over time, given the modest amount of hepatic glycogen stores, most of the tissues (muscle, heart, kidney, etc.) adapt to use mainly fatty acids, saving glucose. The latter will be destined above all to the brain and anaerobic tissues such as red blood cells which, in order to "survive", absolutely need glucose. In fact, they cannot use fatty acids for energy purposes. Under similar conditions, the cerebral demands for glucose amount to 4 g/hour, while those of the anaerobic tissues amount to 1.5 g/hour. Since the liver cannot obtain more than 3g of glucose per hour from glycogenolysis, it is forced to activate an "emergency" metabolic pathway, called gluconeogenesis.

This process consists in the production of glucose starting from amino acids.

Fasting of medium duration
If food deprivation lasts beyond 24 hours, the action described in the adaptation phase continues with a progressive accentuation of gluconeogenesis. The amino acids necessary to satisfy this process derive from the breakdown of muscle proteins. Since there are no protein deposits in the body to be used for energy purposes, the body, in order to survive the fast, is forced to "cannibalize" its muscles. This process is accompanied by an inevitable reduction in muscle mass, with the consequent appearance of weakness and apathy.

In the early stages, gluconeogenesis is capable of producing over 100g of glucose per day, but soon enough the efficiency of this process decreases to around 75 g/day. Unlike what happens during the first phase, this quantity is no longer sufficient to ensure an adequate supply of glucose to the brain. Therefore, this organ is forced to increasingly resort to ketone bodies, three water-soluble molecules deriving from the oxidation of fats in conditions of glucose deficiency. The overproduction of ketone bodies (a process called ketosis), while prolonging the survival of the organism by a few days, causes an important increase in blood acidity.

During fasting periods of medium duration, which extends up to the twenty-fourth day of food deprivation, the recourse of other tissues to lipid oxidation increases more and more, with a general view of maximum saving of blood glucose.

Prolonged fasting and death
This phase begins when the fast lasts beyond the 24th day. The body has now exploited all the protein resources, including plasma proteins. The mix of ketosis, the lowering of the immune defenses, the dehydration and the reduced respiratory efficiency (given by the catabolism of the proteins of the diaphragm and intercostal muscles) condemns the individual to an unfortunate fate.

So should you be afraid of fasting? That's a reasonable question and if you bought this book is because you are interested in seeing what it can do to help you lose weight. Let's be clear from the start: no, fasting is a great solution to burn fat and get healthier. However, there are some important things to point out to avoid making bad mistakes that can result in health damages.

Many people resort to fasting driven by fashions, advertising or food and health beliefs that are at least questionable. Voluntary abstinence from food intake is understood, in these cases, as a moment of physical purification, aimed at eliminating toxins accumulated due to an incorrect diet.

To analyze this fact, after having broadly described the biochemical aspects, we can start from two assumptions. The first, irrefutable, is that we have plenty of food available, a high-calorie food that is often the basis of obesity; in short, we eat too much and the consequences are there for everyone to see. In fact, overeating and a sedentary lifestyle are among the very first causes of death in industrialized countries, including the US. The second point is that a moderately low-calorie diet, summarized in the Japanese saying "hara hachi bu" (get up from the table with an 80% full stomach), is one of the best strategies for living longer and healthier.

While many people should cut down on their food intake, there is no need to resort to extreme solutions such as prohibitive diets or fasting. Instead, it is enough, as our grandparents used to say, to get up from the table when you are still a little hungry and keep in mind that a little exercise never hurts.

Fasting, similar to physical activity, is a stress for the body. The difference is that, while sport leads to an improvement in organic abilities, fasting moves in the opposite direction. The lack and prolonged intake of nutrients reduces muscle mass and basal metabolism (up to 40% in extreme cases). Furthermore, the mind becomes cloudy and a global state of debilitation arises, characterized by a decrease in muscle strength and ability to concentrate. All this has nothing therapeutic or detoxifying.

Partial or attenuated fasting, on the other hand, could have positive implications, as long as it is applied rationally. After a Christmas dinner, for example, it is useful to follow a low-calorie diet rich in liquids and vegetables for two or three days. The important thing is to associate these foods with a certain amount of proteins, perhaps obtained from lean fish (which is usually easy to digest), and fats, for example by consuming a handful of dried fruit. In this way you avoid "cannibalizing your muscles" and depressing your metabolism excessively and then paying the consequences. This last point must also be clear to those who resort to fasting in extremis to lose weight before summer. In fact, a few pounds can be lost but the amount of energy associated with each unit of weight lost is very low. In other words, weight loss is mainly linked to increased diuresis and muscle catabolism induced by prolonged fasting.

As you might have noticed, even if this book is about intermittent fasting for weight loss, we are not advocating the use of fasting without pointing out the importance of doing things the proper way. In fact, the main reason we decided to write this book is to share the right information that can actually make a difference when starting out with intermittent fasting. Your health is extremely important and we would never advise you to do extreme things just to lose a few pounds.

Now that we are done with this disclaimer, we can finally focus on how you can use intermittent fasting to start losing fat.

Chapter 2 - The Basics of Nutrition

We feel it is important to start every diet related book by giving an introduction to the basics of nutrition. In fact, our experience tells us that most people that want to lose weight, do not even know how their body works and what that weight consists of. By having a clear understanding of the two most important elements of nutrition, macronutrients and micronutrients, you are much more likely to conduct a diet that is both healthy and efficient.

Intermittent fasting makes no exception and our focus for the next few pages will be to give you a complete overview of these two macro elements of nutrition.

Macronutrients

Macronutrients are food ingredients that must be introduced in large quantities, as they represent the most important energy source for the body. Carbohydrates, fats (more correctly lipids) and proteins belong to this category. Some scientists include ethyl alcohol in the group of macronutrients; in reality, despite the high caloric value, this substance cannot be considered as such, as it is superfluous for metabolic purposes and devoid of any nutritional value. The attribution of the adjective "macronutrient" to water is more sensible, which however, having a zero calorific value, should simply be considered a food.

Whatever the nutritional plan undertaken, the three macronutrients must always appear in percentage and qualitatively correct quantities.

In the diet of a teetotaler, macronutrients together cover 100% of the total caloric intake and, broadly speaking, about 90% of the dry food weight. In reference to carbohydrates alone, an adult individual consumes a hundred kilos of carbs per year.

All three macronutrients provide energy to the body, but in different quantities and in different biochemical ways.

The proteins, which have a mainly plastic function, provide the organism with materials for the growth, maintenance and reconstruction of cellular structures. Their calorific value is 4Kcal per gram. Carbohydrates - which provide directly available energy - also have a calorific value of 4 Kcal per gram. Lipids, on the other hand, release their energy more slowly, but contain it in concentrations that are more than double (9 Kcal per gram); for this reason, they are particularly important during rest and fasting periods.

Now let's take a closer look at some of the most important macronutrients there are.

Vegetable proteins

Vegetable proteins are amino acid chains with specific biological functions but contained exclusively in cereals, legumes, pseudocereals, vegetables, fruit and oil seeds.

Before talking about vegetable proteins in detail, let's review some very important concepts to establish the quality of a protein source.

Important terms you should know

- Biological value. It represents the quantity of nitrogen actually absorbed and used net of urinary and faecal losses. The reference protein is that of the egg which has a VB equal to 100%

- Protein efficiency ratio (PER). It indicates weight gain in grams for each gram of protein ingested (3.1 for milk; 2.1 for soy)

- Digestibility (D). It is the ratio between ingested and absorbed nitrogen (in descending order wheat, milk and soy).

- Essential Amino Acids (AAE). The term essential indicates the body's inability to synthesize these amino acids from other amino acids through biochemical transformations. There are 20 amino acids involved in protein synthesis and among these 20, only eight are essential (leucine, isoleucine and valine (BCAA), lysine, methionine, threonine, phenylalanine, tryptophan). During the first few years, two other amino acids, arginine and histidine become essential as well.

- Chemical Index. It is found by calculating the ratio between the quantity of a given amino acid in one gram of the protein under examination and the quantity of the same amino acid in one gram of the biological reference protein (of the egg). The higher this index, the greater the percentage of essential amino acids.

Protein quality

In general, the protein quality of foods of animal origin is superior as they contain all the various essential amino acids. The lower quality of vegetable proteins is instead due to a lack of one or more essential amino acids. This amino acid is called the limiting amino acid.

Cereals, for example, are deficient in tryptophan and lysine, an essential amino acid whose deficiency can lead to a deficiency of vitamin B3 (niacin). Legumes, very rich in decent quality proteins, are instead lacking in sulfur amino acids (methionine and cysteine) important for the growth of hair and nails, and for the synthesis of glutathione, a powerful antioxidant able to protect our cells from oxidative stress (free radicals).

However, by correctly combining different vegetable proteins, even alternating ones and not necessarily in the same meal, it is possible to compensate for the lack of various limiting amino acids. In this case we speak of mutual integration (or protein complementation).

Pasta and legumes is an example of an excellent combination since the amino acids that pasta is lacking are supplied by beans and vice versa.

In any case, it should be noted that all the concepts expressed so far must be interpreted rationally.

- If it is true that vegetable proteins are deficient in some amino acids, it does not mean that these are not sufficient to cover the body's protein needs.
- If it is true that limiting amino acids prevent the optimal use of other amino acids for protein synthesis, it does not mean that in these cases the protein synthesis is heavily compromised.
- If it is true that the lack of combination of vegetable proteins can cause protein deficiencies in the long run, this is not valid in the short term. For example, if we dissociate cereals and legumes into two separate meals, the body is perfectly capable of regulating protein synthesis by implementing the limiting amino acids with those present in the endogenous reserves. If, on the other hand, only one type of vegetable protein is consumed for long periods of time (for

example only cereals), the free amino acid stocks are "exhausted" and a protein deficiency inevitably occurs (negative nitrogen balance).

Therefore there are no particular contraindications in consuming mainly food of plant origin as it happens during the summer period. However, it is important that the diet includes the consumption of a wide class of foods of plant origin (dried fruit, vegetables, legumes, etc.) but also of some animal foods (eggs, milk, meats, etc.). In fact, an exclusively vegetarian diet, even if sufficient from a protein point of view, could be deficient in vitamins (B12) and minerals such as iodine, iron and calcium, and essential fatty acids.

Fats
Fats, also called lipids (from the Greek lipos = fat) are a heterogeneous group of substances that have in common a low degree of solubility in water. Instead, they are soluble in organic solvents such as benzene, ether or chloroform.

They are found mainly in foods of animal origin but are also abundantly present in the vegetable kingdom (oils).

Oils and fats are very similar chemically but, while the former are liquid at room temperature, the latter are solid.

There are more than 500 types of fats, classified according to their molecular structure into simple, compound and derivative. Let's take a closer look at their distinction.

- **Simple lipids.** They are the most abundant in our body (about 95%) and in our diet (about 98% of the lipids present in food are ingested in this form). They represent the main form of storage and use. Among the best known are waxes and triglycerides.

- **Compound lipids.** They are triglycerides combined with other chemicals such as phosphorus, nitrogen and sulfur. They represent about 10% of our body's fats. Among the best known are phospholipids, glycolipids and lipoproteins.

- **Lipids derivatives.** They derive from the transformation of simple or compound lipids. The most important is cholesterol, but we also remember vitamin D, steroid hormones, palmitic, oleic and linoleic acid.

Triglycerides derive from the union of a glycerol molecule with three fatty acids in turn formed by hydrocarbon chains ranging from a minimum of 4 to a maximum of 20 carbon atoms.

Triglycerides represent the storage form of fatty acids, a bit like glycogen and glucose. During the energy processes our body in fact breaks down the bond between glycerol and fatty acids, conveying them in two completely different metabolic pathways.

While glycerol is used to produce glucose, free fatty acids are transported into the bloodstream in association with albumin, a plasma protein that carries them to the muscles where they constitute the energy substrate for oxidative processes.

Fats are normally stored by our body as energy and are the building blocks of your belly. By following an intermittent fasting regimen you make sure to burn it away while keeping a good level of health.

Carbohydrates

Carbohydrates, also known as carbs in the fitness world (from the Greek "glucos" = sweet) are substances made up of carbon and water. They have this molecular form: (CH_2O), and are mainly contained in foods of plant origin.

On average they provide 4 kcal per gram, even if their energy value fluctuates from 3.74 kcal of glucose to 4.2 Kcal of starch. About 10% of these calories is used by the body for digestion and absorption processes.

Based on their chemical structure, carbohydrates are classified into simple and complex.

Simple carbohydrates, commonly called sugars, include monosaccharides, disaccharides and oligosaccharides. In nature there are more than 200 monosaccharides which differ in the number of carbon atoms present in their chain.

Hexoses (fructose, glucose, galactose) are the most important from a nutritional point of view. Let's take a look at the different types of carbs there are.

Monosaccharides
- Glucose is normally found in foods, both in free form and in the form of polysaccharide. It constitutes the

form in which the other sugars must be transformed in order to be used by our body. Only 5% of the total amount of carbohydrates present in our body is represented by glucose circulating in the blood. Glycemic index = 100.

- Fructose is found in abundance in fruit and honey; it is absorbed in the small intestine and metabolized by the liver which transforms it into glucose. Its glycemic index is very low, equal to 23.
- Galactose in nature is not found free but it is always linked to glucose it forms lactose, the sugar of milk.

Oligosaccharides are formed by the union of two or more monosaccharides (maximum 10). They are found mainly in vegetables and in particular in legumes. The best known, since they are important from a nutritional point of view are disaccharides (sucrose, lactose and maltose).

Disaccharides

- Sucrose. Glucose + fructose; very common in nature it is present in honey, beets and sugar cane. Its glycemic index is 68 ± 5.

- Lactose. Glucose + galactose; it is the sugar of milk and the least sweet of the disaccharides. Its glycemic index is 46 ± 6.
- Maltose. Little present in our diet is found mainly in beer, cereals and sprouts. Its glycemic index is 109.

Among the oligosaccharides we mention maltodextrins.

Oligosaccharides

Maltodextrins are oligosaccharides deriving from the hydrolysis process of starches. They are used as energy supplements and can be useful in endurance sports. They provide short and medium term energy without straining the digestive system too much.

Polysaccharides are formed by the union of numerous monosaccharides (from 10 to thousands) through glycosidic bonds. Vegetable polysaccharides (starches and fibers) and polysaccharides of animal origin (glycogen) are distinguished. Polysaccharides containing a single type of sugar are called homopolysaccharides, while those containing different types of monosaccharides are called heteropolysaccharides.

Polysaccharides

- Starch is the carbohydrate reserve of vegetables. It abounds in seeds, cereals; it is also found in large quantities in peas, beans and sweet potatoes. It occurs naturally in two forms, amylose and amylopectin. The higher the amylopectin content, the more digestible the food is.

- Fibers are structural polysaccharides, the most important of which is cellulose. Our body is not able to use them for energy purposes, but their fermentation in the intestine is essential to regulate the absorption of nutrients and to protect our body from numerous diseases. They are divided into water-soluble and non-water-soluble. The former chelate by interfering with the absorption of nutrients, including cholesterol, the latter attract water, accelerating gastric emptying. The caloric contribution of fiber in the diet is zero.

- Glycogen is a polysaccharide similar to amylopectin used as a source of storage and primary energy reserve. It is stored in the liver and muscles up to a maximum of 400-500 grams. The glycogen present in animals is almost completely degraded at the time of slaughter so it is present in extremely small quantities in food.

In general, carbohydrates can be considered an easy to access source of energy. Most athletes take them before training as they give your body immediate energy to perform activities. When doing intermittent fasting, you want to avoid eating carbohydrates during the fasting periods as your goal is to empty the glycogen in your muscles to start burning fat.

Micronutrients

Vitamins and Minerals are nutrients that do not bring energy, but whose presence is essential for the correct functioning of the organism. They work at very low doses and are therefore referred to as micronutrients.

For people in general, but especially for athletes, microelements can make the difference in sports training;

especially for bodybuilders, who often fail to meet their needs for the following reasons.

- Some have milk intolerance and do not eat dairy products due to the fat content.
- Many do not eat vegetables or fruit due to their sugar content or because they are not very pleasing to the palate.
- They consume minimal amounts of fat and not at every meal.
- In pre-competition diets they almost totally eliminate fats and carbohydrates.

It follows that integration is almost always indispensable for these people.

For example, for minerals it would be useful to carry out a blood test or a hair analysis to see if you have a deficiency or not. Most women over 50 tend to suffer from this type of deficiency and we advise you to consult your doctor to see if a supplement can help you out. Another option would be to take a multivitamin-mineral complex daily, you cannot go wrong with it. Some vitamins have a very short life (especially the water-soluble ones, which only last 3-4 hours) so it is better to use a prolonged release compound associated, perhaps, with essential fatty acids.

Vitamins

They are enzymatic substances and, similar to some amino acids and fatty acids, they are essential nutrients, as our body is unable to synthesize them. The vitamin requirement varies greatly from one individual to another, because the activity of certain enzymes can differ up to 50 times from case to case. Depending on their solubility we distinguish the vitamins into fat-soluble and water-soluble.

The fat-soluble vitamins are stored in the body and can give rise to overdosing phenomena. If, on the other hand, one or more of these substances, whether or not they are soluble in water, are supplied in insufficient quantities, deficiency problems arise. We will therefore talk about avitaminosis and hypovitaminosis.

Avitaminosis is the complete lack of a vitamin; while this problem is rare in countries in good economic conditions, it is a common plague in underdeveloped regions. Much more widespread than one might believe, even in industrialized populations, is hypovitaminosis, that is, the partial lack of vitamins; the causes are mainly found in the high consumption of preserved foods, as well as artificially ripened fruit and vegetables. Furthermore, vitamin deficiencies may arise due to the administration of drugs, especially antibiotics or due to increased needs during pregnancy, breastfeeding, growth, infectious diseases and intense physical activity.

As we already mentioned, most women over 50 are highly recommended to supplement their diet with a good multivitamin-mineral complex. Go to your local drug store and you will certainly find someone able to advise you on the best one for you.

Minerals

A mineral is a substance made up of the combination of a metallic and a non-metallic element. These "elements" are "simple bodies" that are not divisible. The universe is made up of 103 known chemical elements, of which 22 are indispensable for the organism; others are present in traces but are not essential. On the contrary, they can even become toxic, such as arsenium, mercury or lead, to the point of causing death.

These elements cannot be created or destroyed, but they are preserved integrally and cannot be transformed to cover a deficiency.

Hydrogen is the basic element from which all others are composed. In fact, 96% of the human body is made up of only 4 elements:

- oxygen;
- carbon;
- hydrogen;
- nitrogen

Oxygen represents 65% of body weight. The remaining 4% is composed of the other elements, of which 2.5% (of the total body weight) is given by calcium and phosphorus.

The chemical composition varies from individual to individual and depends on different aspects as we will see in a minute. For example a bodybuilder will have a higher nitrogen percentage than that of a normal individual. There can be significant differences in the content of mineral elements between various individuals, due to the following reasons.

- Age. Many metallic elements tend to accumulate over the years and it is not a surprise that women over 50 have a greater mineral concentration than younger people.

- Sex. Men and women have a different concentration of minerals in their bodies.

- Physical activity. A more active person tends to accumulate more minerals, especially if supplements are taken on a regular basis.

- Drugs. People that take drugs on a regular basis tend to accumulate more minerals. The higher concentration can be due to past events as well, especially if the drugs were strong.

- Eating habits. Minerals are generally found in high quality fruits and vegetables. If you conduct a healthy intermittent fasting lifestyle you should not have any issue concerning minerals.

- The environment. Certain regions are richer in terms of minerals present in the soil. Clearly, everything that is cultivated in these places will have greater minerals concentration as well.

The origin of the food is fundamental. In fact, if a certain element is not present in the soil it will not be present in the fruits and vegetables that are cultivated there. Furthermore, they will not be present in high concentration in the meat of the animals that feed in that place as well. In theory, in order to have all the foods we need, we would have to eat everything at every meal, but this is practically impossible. Furthermore, for the correct assimilation of minerals the presence of vitamins is often necessary and vice versa. Many minerals to be active must be linked to other substances and the fat-soluble vitamins require the simultaneous presence of fats. Finally, excessive consumption of alcohol and dietary fiber can create intestinal malabsorption problems.

Considering that most of the water-soluble vitamins are eliminated within a few hours, the ideal would be to take a small amount of a multivitamin-mineral supplement with each meal. Once again, your local drug store will have everything you need. Go and ask for advice!

We can divide minerals into macroelements that are present in the organism in greater quantities and into oligoelements, that are present in infinitesimal quantities. Among the latter we still have some useful elements (zinc, iron, iodine, selenium, manganese, copper) and some toxic elements, such as lead, mercury, cadmium and arsenic. In any case, the toxicity of minerals essentially depends on the amount that is consumed by the body. This means they are all potentially toxic at high doses.

We hope that by reading this chapter you have understood the importance and the complexity of nutrition. It is a fascinating topic that could last for many more pages. However, our goal was to give you the basic concepts and help you realize that when it comes to intermittent fasting is not just a matter of not eating for a certain period of time. You have to know what to eat after your fasting as well, as your body will need to be fed properly after such a stressful event.

Especially if you are a woman over 50, we advise you to pay particular attention to your eating habits after fasting. They are what can make or break your ability to lose weight and, most importantly, be healthy. When in doubt, consult a professional doctor.

Chapter 3 - Benefits of Intermittent Fasting

Now that we have discussed the basics of nutrition, let's begin our journey into the fascinating world of intermittent fasting by taking a look at the benefits it has.

Intermittent fasting is a weight loss system based on the cardinal principle of creating a window of fasting with a duration that affects the overall caloric balance and hormonal metabolism. In conditions of food abstinence, in addition to a total insulin calm (remember that insulin is the anabolic hormone par excellence but also responsible for adipose deposition), there is a significant increase in another hormone: IGF-1 or somatomedin (some even mention an increase in testosterone). The intermittent deprivation of food is then responsible for the secretion of GH (somatotropin), known as the "feel-good hormone". Unlike insulin, GH, while increasing hypertrophy, does not cause fat deposits, but favors the lipolysis necessary for weight loss and muscle definition.

The main dietary regimes that involve intermittent fasting are the following three.

- Fasting every other day;
- Fasting for 2 days a week;
- Daily fasting (the period of the day during which the individual eats is limited to 8-12 hours and the remaining 12-14-16 hours are dedicated to fasting).

Dietary pattern of intermittent fasting
The food pattern of intermittent fasting consists of 3 daily meals and 1 training session with a fasting window of 16 hours. This is what experts recommend to women over 50 that are starting this eating regiment.

This is a quick scheme of a typical intermittent fasting day.

- 1st meal to be consumed as soon as you get up. For this first meal, a protein and carbohydrates source with a medium-low glycemic index is advised. Please, avoid consuming high fat foods in this first meal.

- 2nd meal. This should be your breakfast. In this case, eat a complete meal high in macronutrients and micronutrients. Take your supplements during this meal.

- Training. We will have a dedicated chapter to training for women of your age, but in this case a light bodybuilding routing or high intensity training should be a good indication.

- 3rd meal. Consume this immediately after training. This is your lunch, so make sure you eat your carbs, proteins and fats.

- Fasting window from about 1:00 pm or 3:00 pm until the following morning.

Benefits of intermittent fasting

Some specialists propose to treat overweight and metabolic diseases through the so-called therapeutic fasting. This practice takes place under conditions of medical supervision and nutritional support. Fasting can be beneficial or harmful based on some factors: duration, completeness of food abstention, pathological conditions for its application, etc.

Not all forms of fasting are created equal. In fact, some are extremely debilitating and harmful, others are less exhausting and more rational.

Several studies have highlighted the body's health benefits of intermittent fasting. Not only weight loss and the contrast of free radicals, which translated can seem like an elixir of life, but also resources capable of regulating blood sugar levels and inflammation. From a cardiovascular health perspective, intermittent fasting improves blood pressure levels, resting heart rate, blood triglyceride and cholesterol levels, and reduces oxidative stress related to the development of atherosclerosis.

Effects on metabolism

As we have seen in the previous chapter, the main essential nutrients for our body are sugars (especially glucose), proteins and fatty acids. After meals, excess fats are accumulated in the adipose tissue in the form of triglycerides which are broken down into glycerol and fatty acids during fasting. The liver converts fatty acids into ketone bodies, which provide energy to many organs. During intermittent fasting the levels of ketone bodies increase in the blood of humans approximately 8-12 hours after the last meal is consumed. The change in metabolism affects the regulation of glucose levels, blood pressure, heart rate and abdominal fat loss.

Effects on health and aging

Caloric restriction (i.e. the reduction of food intake) seems to increase life expectancy. In some studies, people subjected to intermittent fasting have shown the following positive results.

- weight loss;
- reduction in abdominal circumference;
- better insulin sensitivity and therefore a lower risk of developing diabetes;
- greater muscle endurance;
- increased cognitive ability.

However, there is a lack of scientific validation capable of defining whether these effects are related to intermittent fasting or to the caloric deficit alone.

The Okinawa case

The island of Okinawa (south of Japan) holds the absolute record for the number of ultra-centennial inhabitants. Here intermittent fasting is practiced regularly, mainly vegetables, seaweed, goya, tofu, fish (very raw, even large pieces such as tuna) and very little meat are eaten. Another very important aspect that characterizes the eating style of the inhabitants of this Japanese island is caloric moderation; in this regard, a famous local saying suggests eating about 80% of the food needed to feel full. We truly agree with this philosophy of life. You should never become enslaved to your food.

Long-term applicability
Despite the disparate health benefits of intermittent fasting, incorporating this practice into everyday life is not easy. In fact, during the first few weeks, most people have to deal with anger, irritability, and difficulty concentrating. Before starting intermittent fasting it is necessary to ask for the help of a nutritionist or dietician to ensure a balanced intake of macro and micro nutrients. Once again, we remind you that this book is for entertainment purposes only and we advise you to see medical help before starting any diet.

Chapter 4 - Therapeutic Fasting

In the previous chapter we mentioned the possibility to use fasting to cure some pathologies. Since the goal of this book is to give you every tool and information you might need to develop a healthy lifestyle through intermittent fasting, we feel it is our duty to dedicate a chapter to this important subject. The last thing we want is to have people with severe conditions reading this book and thinking they can just fast them away.

In nature, because food is not always available, intermittent fasting is part of the survival routine and any animal organism can handle it.

For humans, fasting means refraining from consuming some or all foods, drinks or both, for a period of time that can be determined or indefinite.

Absolute fasting is defined as the failure to eat any solid or liquid food for a certain period, usually between 24 hours or more than a few days.

Imposed Fast

For evolutionary reasons, the human body (thanks to its hormonal flows) is able to adapt optimally to the absence of food. The same cannot be said for overeating, as a result of which you can get sick of the so-called diseases of well-being (obesity, dyslipidemia, type 2 diabetes mellitus, hypertension, etc.).

In this regard, some specialists propose to treat overweight and metabolic diseases through the so-called therapeutic fasting. This practice takes place under conditions of medical supervision and nutritional support (with food supplements and water taken on a regular basis).

As we have seen in previous chapters as well, fasting can be beneficial or harmful based on some factors. For example: duration, completeness of food abstention or nutritional support, medical control, pathological conditions for its application, etc.

Fasting, whether controlled or uncontrolled, therapeutic or not, is still very stressful for the body and mind. However, its potential harmfulness mainly depends on the parameters with which it is programmed.

An example of highly questionable fasting is the so-called tube diet. This is based on a form of chronic fasting, during which the body is supported exclusively by enteral artificial nutrition (nasogastric tube).

We do not endorse these types of fasting. In fact, similar practices can have the following consequences.

- Physical debility and tendency to malnutrition and ketosis;
- Limitation of physical activities;
- Food miseducation.

On the contrary, in subjects suffering from metabolic pathologies, short periods of food interruption - such as, for example, the emphasis on the night fasting period (that during sleep, taking it from 8 to 12 or 14 hours) - does not cause side effects. and favor the remission of certain metabolic parameters (especially hyperglycemia and hypertriglyceridemia) or other disorders (fatty liver, gastroesophageal reflux, etc.). Obviously, the example just reported does not represent a real fast and this is the only form of food abstention potentially beneficial and free of side effects.

Many believe that absolute fasting can negatively affect hormonal flows, specifically by suppressing the action of the thyroid gland (the one that secretes the hormones responsible for regulating metabolism); this is only partially true. In fact, prolonged fasting undoubtedly reduces the secretion of thyroid hormones. However, in general, this reduction does not occur before 24 or 48 hours.

There is some scientific evidence showing that fasting can play an important role in people receiving chemotherapy, but more studies are needed to define its actual efficacy and possible clinical application.

Can fasting be used to cure some conditions?

Some centers specialized in the treatment of metabolic diseases use therapeutic fasting for weight reduction and for the restoration of metabolic parameters.

Therapeutic fasting systems rarely rely on irrevocable abstinence from food, and none of these prohibit the use of water. On the contrary, the tendency is to encourage the intake of liquids and, sometimes, of certain plant foods in certain portions (especially in the case of certain particular diseases).

According to the experience of the operators who propose therapeutic fasting, the greatest difficulty consists in the initial acceptance of the therapy, not in the protocol itself. Few believe people can survive 2 or 3 weeks without eating but, on the other hand, many have spontaneously reached 30-40 days.

How does it work?
The first 24-48 hours of therapy include complete fasting with the sole intake of water.

In this phase, which is also the hardest, the body consumes most of the sugar and triglycerides present in the blood. Obviously, glucose levels are kept progressively stable by hepatic glycogen, while motor action (typified by absolute rest) is mainly supported by muscle glycogen stores.

Warning! As of now, it is already quite clear that this technique cannot be used in the case of liver impairment, type 1 diabetes or other diseases that involve significant metabolic difficulty.

The true metabolic action (or rather, that sought by therapists) occurs at the end of this first phase, that is when the glycogen reserves are reduced to the bone. At this point, the body begins to burn mainly the adipose tissue, with the production and blood flow of molecules called ketones.

Sometimes, in compromised subjects or those who take certain drugs, therapeutic fasting involves the intake of vegetable juices to reduce the state of ketoacidosis.

Therapeutic fasting is interrupted in progressive matters, starting with the intake of juices and centrifuged, then of smoothies and vegetable cut in small pieces, reaching up to the intake of cereals and legumes.

Effects

Ketones, although potentially toxic, can have positive effects on therapeutic compliance. This depends on the tolerance of the patient.

In fact, by acting in a suppressive manner against the central nervous system, ketones reduce the stimulus of hunger to a minimum.

Some even claim that ketones can cause a feeling of general well-being. However, this condition called "ketoacidosis" is not free from side effects, including: liver and kidney toxicity, tendency to dehydration, hypotension, and many other conditions you need to avoid.

Fasting and digestive rest

Those who propose therapeutic fasting affirm that this feeling of well-being is not attributable only to ketoacidosis, but also to the total rest of the gastrointestinal tract.

Indeed, the digestion of subjects suffering from obesity is always a rather demanding process. In fact, by consuming very abundant meals, not very digestible and responsible for high glycemic peaks, these people are used to living with a feeling of almost continuous psycho-physical weakness.

Fasting and cell washing
A further beneficial effect of therapeutic fasting, further emphasized by the administration of antioxidant supplements, is the so-called cell washing. Not everyone knows that the organism has various means of excretion of useless or toxic molecules; among these we find the following:
- bile
- feces
- urine
- sweat
- mucus
- lung ventilation

- hair
- nails

Therapeutic fasting makes it possible to exploit these mechanisms without simultaneously taking in other pollutants or other toxic agents, among which we remember: mercury, arsenic, lead, dioxin and food additives.

Fasting and taste buds

Another great advantage of therapeutic fasting is the restoration of the gustatory papillary function of the tongue, which occurs through a process called neuroadaptation.

This perceptual reset effect of tastes is very useful for the subsequent reorganization of the diet in the maintenance phase, which involves the exclusive use of fresh and lightly seasoned foods.

Recommendations

Therapeutic fasting violates every principle of dietetics and nutritional balance. It is a radical intervention that could find application in the replacement of bariatric surgery.

It must be remembered that ketogenic diets have a very deleterious effect on the body, starting from kidney fatigue up to the wasting of muscle tissue.

Regardless of personal or professional opinion, it is important to underline that it is objectively a technique that can only be practiced within specialized structures, where medical personnel are able to supervise the entire process and, if necessary, implement the use of drugs or specific supplements.

The nutritional supplements, on the other hand, are vitamin, saline and amino acid in nature; the overall advice for those facing therapeutic fasting is to suspend any drug treatment, except for those that cannot be discontinued. In the presence of certain pathologies (organic or psychiatric), of special physiological conditions (pregnancy, breastfeeding), old age and growth, therapeutic fasting is totally not recommended.

We would like to end this chapter by pointing out that intermittent fasting and therapeutic fasting are two totally different things. While therapeutic fasting requires medical supervision during the entire process, a healthy intermittent fasting routine can be conducted autonomously by visiting your doctor once every couple of weeks.

For women of your age we encourage you to seek professional advice before, during and after this practice.

Chapter 5 - Training while Fasting

Training on an empty stomach has a number of undoubted advantages in terms of lipid oxidation, deriving from the metabolic implications of morning hypoglycemia. It is no coincidence that this training technique is now widely used to promote weight loss intended as a loss of fat mass in favor of lean.

Benefits of training while fasting

Running or cycling for 30 minutes early in the morning, after an overnight fast, is one of the most popular practices for weight loss. In fact, it is believed that aerobic activity carried out on an empty stomach allows you to burn greater quantities of superfluous fat, raising the metabolism for the rest of the day and promoting psychophysical well-being. In the morning, due to the long night fast, blood sugar and glycogen stores are generally lower than the rest of the day; given the relative lack of glucose in the blood, training in these conditions promotes a greater use of fat in terms of energy. The hormonal picture is also favorable, characterized by low insulin levels and high levels of counterinsular hormones such as adrenaline, noradrenaline, cortisol, thyroxine, glucagon, and growth hormone. All these hormones promote weight loss by directly or indirectly stimulating lipolysis. The strong adrenergic secretion (adrenaline and noradrenaline) recorded during exercise significantly raises the metabolism, which remains elevated for a certain period even after the end of the training session. The important release of endorphins induced by physical activity is instead potentially useful for promoting the sense of psychophysical well-being for the rest of the day.

Training on an empty stomach, with the intention of losing weight, could lead to excessive muscle catabolism, since in conditions of hypoglycemia the amount of energy obtained from amino acids also increases. Since consuming solid foods or a protein mix would lessen the metabolic benefits induced by fasting, to prevent excessive muscle catabolism it may be helpful to ingest a few branched chain amino tablets before training. For the same reason, in order to avoid excessive protein catabolism, it is advisable not to prolong fasting aerobics beyond 30-40 minutes.

Fasting workouts should be placed in a dietary context aimed at weight loss. The ideal is to combine these aerobic sessions with weight training (obviously at different times of the day) focused on strength development. Be careful though. In fact, this does not mean that you have to train with a high number of repetitions. Rather, demanding loads in perfect short and intense style will be used. This is effective for women of your age as well, not just younger athletes.

Training on an empty stomach increases the risk of hypoglycemic attacks, especially in untrained subjects or those not used to exercising in such conditions; the onset of hypoglycaemia is signaled by symptoms such as craving for food, paleness, cold sweat, headache and dizziness, excessive irritability, tremor, agitation, difficulty concentrating and risk of fainting. At the onset of these symptoms, it is good to stop running immediately. Normally, in these cases the symptoms will then be resolved by taking small amounts of foods rich in sugars (chocolates, dextrose, sweetened soft drinks, honey, raisins), followed by a more substantial meal based on complex carbohydrates. This second meal is consumed to prevent reactive hypoglycemia from copious ingestion of simple sugars.

Taking a couple of coffees or a thermogenic supplement (based on bitter orange, synephrine, mate, guarana, cola, tea, theine or theobromine), before training is theoretically useful to enhance the lipolytic action.

Before starting the workout, it is good to drink a couple of glasses of water, especially when you do not have the opportunity to drink during the training session.

Running while fasting could also induce excessive stress from a psychic point of view, especially when too many hours of night rest are sacrificed. For this reason, this practice is generally limited to those short definition periods that precede a photo shoot, a bodybuilding competition or the arrival of summer. All this also by virtue of the fact that it is not a miraculous strategy, given that the advantages compared to traditional training are limited. On the other hand, in front of a sprinter we notice a lean and muscular body despite his training involving a negligible consumption of fat. This makes us understand, in case the concept is not yet clear, that the ideal physical activity for weight loss cannot be separated from exercises with weights and high intensity isotonic machines. This has to be combined with traditional but often overrated aerobic workouts, independently whether they are carried out on an empty stomach or not.

Even for women of your age, we recommend combining aerobic training with strength training. In the next few chapters we are going to give you a detailed description of the different types of training you can follow in order to lose weight while intermittent fasting.

Please, note how we are putting the discussion of the different training methodologies before the actual fasting programs. That's because we believe that the only way to actually burn fat while maintaining muscle mass when you reach a certain age is to implement a consistent training program.

In this book we have decided to give you two options for aerobic training and one option for strength training. Let's see them in detail.

Chapter 6 - Intermittent Fasting and Aerobic Training

Physical activity, if practiced consistently and following the correct directions, can bring significant benefits both physically and mentally. Recent studies have shown that aerobic training is even miraculous for our body and to improve our mental state.

What is aerobic training?

Aerobic training or better known by the term "cardio" is widely practiced in the gym and differs from anaerobic training in the manner, timing and intensity with which the exercises are carried out. Aerobic training is done with an intensity that allows our body to use carbohydrates and fats as fuel. When an aerobic workout takes place, the body "draws" energy from the reserves of sugars and fat deposits, thus increasing energy expenditure and promoting weight loss as well. Aerobic training does not take place for long periods of time, but for a maximum of 20-30 consecutive minutes and the intensity of sports activity has normal and well-defined rhythms, not as intense and prolonged as in anaerobic activities. In carrying out an aerobic activity, a small amount of lactic acid is produced, so as not to cause sudden changes or peaks in the heart rate and always maintaining a constant and fairly consistent rhythm. The main aerobic activities that can be practiced are the following.

- cycling;
- running;
- spinning;
- boxing;
- functional training;
- cross-country skiing.

Other team sports such as table tennis or other activities that can be practiced in the gym can also be included in the list of aerobic activities.

The benefits of aerobic training
Aerobic training is important for those who want to obtain specific benefits for the body and mind. Let's see together which are the main ones. Aerobic activity can be associated with cardiovascular training. In fact, one of the main benefits

of practicing this type of activity is to improve the entire circulatory system. In particular, during aerobic training, it is possible to use a greater amount of oxygen, thus helping to improve blood circulation. The benefits for the cardio-circulatory system are not only for the heart, but there has been a significant improvement in vascular function and in blood pressure parameters.

Aerobic training also brings significant benefits to the respiratory system. In fact, many scientific studies have shown that greater tissue oxygenation is obtained after practicing aerobic sports. At the respiratory level, aerobic activity improves the elasticity and functioning of the pulmonary alveoli, reducing the presence of elements harmful to the health of the organism.

With cardio training the absorption of calcium is facilitated. In this way the bones are strengthened and the muscles become more flexible and elastic. Aerobic activity, since it brings significant benefits to bones and joints, is particularly suitable for women over 50 that want to prevent the onset of bone diseases. A recent study conducted by the University of Illinois has shown how cardio training helps improve the immune system, reducing the attack of bacteria and viruses that cause colds or flu.

The advantages of choosing a cardio workout are not only physical, but several mental benefits have been highlighted by recent studies as well. Like every physical activity, aerobic efforts also help to improve general mood: during training, the body produces oxytocin, better known as the hormone of happiness, thus promoting relaxation and lowering stress levels. Aerobic training is particularly recommended for people suffering from depression or for those suffering from generalized anxiety. Among the advantages of practicing an aerobic activity, there is also that of being able to play sports in the open air, favoring breathing and relaxation.

The main differences between aerobic and anaerobic training

When it comes to aerobic and anaerobic training, it is necessary to highlight what the main differences between these two types of physical activity are. Aerobic training mostly consists in the repetition of exercises for a prolonged period of time, performed with a fairly moderate effort, without sudden variations. Anaerobic training, on the other hand, is carried out by performing short-duration exercises for a limited period of time, but employing greater effort.

The differences between aerobic and anaerobic training do not only concern the way in which the exercises are performed, but also how the body responds to these stimuli. In fact, aerobic training draws energy from sugar and fat stores, while anaerobic training draws it from sugar reserves, muscles and liver, so that you have to stop exercising after a few minutes to allow the body to restore the energy consumed. During aerobic training there is a large production of lactic acid, while in cardio, the production of lactic acid is limited. The two types of training produce different effects on the body. In fact, those who practice aerobic activity tend to lose weight fast, while those who exercise anaerobically increase muscle mass and strengthen certain parts of the body.

This is the reason why we recommend to implement both of them for reaching a great level of wellbeing.

How aerobic training can help weight loss
Cardio training is particularly suitable for those women who want to lose weight. In fact, if combined with a balanced intermittent fasting regimen, it can help you lose excess pounds with ease.

Aerobic activity is by definition fat burning at its finest. In fact by drawing on the fat storage reserves, it accelerates metabolism and promotes weight loss, and also helps to decrease cholesterol and triglyceride levels. For example, jogging allows you to slim your body and make your legs leaner, but at the same time it tones and makes your muscles and joints more flexible. Swimming, which has always been considered a "complete" sport, allows you to lose weight and lose excess pounds and at the same time improve flexibility, endurance and muscle tone.

What to eat after aerobic training
Many people, after having performed an aerobic activity outdoors or in the gym, do not want to risk compromising their efforts by consuming too much caloric food. If you train early in the morning, you need to have a fruit-based snack before starting your workout. We recommend you a banana, mango and cocoa-based smoothie, while snacks and coffee are to be avoided.
To restore energy after an aerobic workout, it is necessary to consume mainly carbohydrates and limit the intake of proteins. In particular, for a post-workout lunch or dinner you can have legumes, wholemeal pasta and cereals, but not in excessive quantities. In combination with carbohydrates, you can consume lean chicken and turkey meat and as

always fruit and vegetables are the best foods if you want to keep your vitamins high.

Now that we have discussed the basics of aerobic training, we would like to give you a little training program for two aerobic activities you can do without too much equipment. First of all, we are going to provide you with an easy to follow running program that will get you started even if you have never run a mile in your life. Secondly, we will explain how you can implement cycling with intermittent fasting. In particular, we recommend you to choose cycling over running if you have joint problems, as it is less stressful for your body.

Intermittent fasting and running

As we mentioned before, we advise you to go for your aerobic activity before eating. If you will decide to follow our basic intermittent fasting program (more on that in the next chapters), this means you will run in the morning. On the other hand, if you go with our more advanced fasting program (once again, more on that later), you will go for a run before lunch.

In both these scenarios you can follow this easy running program to start from zero and work your way up to 5km (3.1 Miles) in one running session.

The program is on the next page.

	Week 1	Week 2	Week 3	Week 4	Week 5	Week 6
Monday	5 min walk, 1 min run, 1 min walk (repeat 5 times), 5 min walk	5 min walk, 1 min run, 1 min walk (repeat 5 times), 5 min walk	5 min walk, 2 min run, 1 min walk (repeat 5 times), 5 min walk	5min walk, 5min run, 1min walk (repeat 3 times), 5min walk	5 minutes of walking, 12 minutes of running, 2 minutes of walking, 6 minutes of running, 5 minutes of walking	5 minutes of walking, 16 minutes of running, 2 minutes of walking, 6 minutes of running, 5 minutes of walking
Tuesday	Rest	Rest	Rest	Rest	Rest	Rest
Wednesday	5 min walk, 1 min run, 1 min walk (repeat 5 times), 5 min walk	5 min walk, 1 min run, 1 min walk (repeat 8 times), 5 min walk	5min walk, 3min run, 1min walk (repeat 4 times), 5min walk	5 min walk, 6 min run, 1 min walk (repeat 3 times), 5 min walk	5 minutes of walking, 14 minutes of running, 3 minutes of walking, 6 minutes of running, 5 minutes of walking	5 minutes of walking, 18 minutes of running, 2 minutes of walking, 8 minutes of running, 5 minutes of walking
Thursday	Rest	Rest	Rest	Rest	Rest	Rest
Friday	5 min walk, 1 min run, 1 min walk (repeat 5 times), 5 min walk	5min walk, 1min run, 1min walk (repeat 10 times), 5min walk	5min walk, 4min run, 1min walk (repeat 3 times), 5min walk	5 min walk, 7 min run, 1 min walk (repeat 3 times), 5 min walk	5 minutes of walking, 16 minutes of running, 2 minutes of walking, 7 minutes of running, 5 minutes of walking	5 minutes of walking, 22 minutes of running, 2 minutes of walking, 10 minutes of running, 5 minutes of walking
Saturday	Rest	Rest	Rest	Rest	Rest	Rest

S u n d a y	30min walk	30min walk	10 minutes of walking, 10 minutes of running, 10 minutes of walking	5 minutes of walking, 15 minutes of running, 5 minutes of walking	5 minutes of walking, 25 minutes of running, 5 minutes of walking	5 km (3.1 Miles)

As you can see, the total time per training session is not very long and it almost never goes over 30 minutes. We feel that this is the optimal duration for an aerobic training session for women over 50 years of age, as you want to dedicate more time to strengthen your muscles rather than losing fat. Intermittent fasting will do that for you.

Intermittent fasting and cycling

Before moving on to the anaerobic training programs, let's take a quick look at how you can start cycling. As mentioned before, this is a great physical activity for women of your age that suffer from joints related pain and prefer aerobic efforts that are less stressful for the body.

If you have never used a bicycle before, we recommend you start by following this little program that will get you in shape to go for a ride of 60 minutes. Since cycling burns less calories than running, you will need to train for a longer period of time to burn the same amount.

	Week 1	Week 2	Week 3	Week 4	Week 5	Week 6
Monday	20' ride	25' ride	30' ride	35' ride	40' ride	45' ride
Tuesday	rest	rest	rest	rest	rest	rest
Wednesday	20' ride	25' ride	30' ride	35' ride	40' ride	45' ride
Thursday	rest	rest	rest	rest	rest	rest
Friday	25' ride	30' ride	35' ride	40' ride	40' ride	30' ride
Saturday	30' ride	35' ride	40' ride	45' ride	45' ride	rest
Sunday	rest	rest	rest	rest	rest	60' ride

Now that we have seen how to start cycling even if you have never ridden a bicycle before, we can focus our attention on what type of strength training to perform while following an intermittent fasting regiment. The next chapter will tell you everything about it.

Chapter 7 - Intermittent Fasting and Strength Training

Even though weight training in the gym is no longer an area reserved for men, muscle development and strength training for women are still scary at times. In fact, the fear of getting too muscular and losing female curves is widespread and prevents many women from practicing strength training or weight lifting. In particular, when it comes to losing a few pounds or reducing body fat, strength training is the key to success.

Many movie, music and sports stars practice it and post the results of their favorite workouts or exercises on social networks. In fact, strength training is an indispensable ally for achieving a dream silhouette and these stars know what they have to do to stay in shape.

As a woman over 50 years of age, is it possible to lose weight thanks to strength training?
Let's start from the basics. To lose weight it is essential to reach a caloric deficit. By exercising, you help the weight loss process by increasing your calorie consumption and

maintaining muscle tone. If you additionally do strength exercises, you signal to your body that it still needs to keep the muscles active and in turn it counteracts muscle loss. The consequence is that you lose weight and your body is fitter and more toned.

Aerobic training is not enough
It is often noted that in the gym women mostly use cardio equipment and avoid weights and strength-training tools. But the key to success for having a toned and defined body is strength training.

Muscle mass, which is 22% of the total body mass, consumes almost a quarter of our daily energy balance. Muscles are the most powerful weapon against excess pounds and fat pads. Muscles burn calories even at rest and increase the basal metabolism which stimulates long-term fat burning.

Strength training for women not only serves to develop quality muscle mass, but also contributes to the maintenance of existing muscles. A pure resistance training combined with a low calorie diet allows you to reach the caloric deficit, but in the long term the weight loss also results in loss of muscle mass.

The loss of muscle mass lowers the body's energy needs, which often continues even after weight loss.

The consequences are the following.

- it becomes more and more difficult to reach the calorie deficit and therefore to burn fat;
- after the first few weeks, the risk of the so-called "yoyo effect" is real.

And here comes strength training that helps maintain, defines existing muscles and promotes fat burning. Endurance training is an intelligent integration of strength training. It helps burn additional calories, improve performance and strengthen the cardiovascular system.

Don't be afraid of getting too muscular
The fear of getting too muscular by engaging in weightlifting or strength training is totally unfounded. Women are biologically programmed differently from men. They have the same muscle structure, but typically produce much less testosterone, a hormone that promotes muscle development. The woman's body also differs from the male one in terms of muscle development, strength and fat percentage. For these

reasons, there is no danger of becoming a little cube of muscles, but training will help you acquire a rounded and defined shape.

To stimulate the muscles during training and achieve good definition, you need adequate resistance. Even if you are over 50, do not be afraid to go heavy in the gym. Lift with your heart and use your muscles, they want to be used!

The benefits of strength training for women

Defined and toned shapes are one of the many advantages of strength training for women. The whole body is toned and the muscles are defined, two aspects that make a woman's body more beautiful as well. By increasing the percentage of muscle mass and decreasing fat, the lines are more defined and the feminine curves stand out more.

Unlike aerobic training, in strength training you can train individual muscles or muscle groups, thus modeling certain parts of the body.

The proportions of the body can therefore be changed, creating a more harmonious silhouette. For example, a large pelvis can be balanced by training and developing the upper body. In addition, strength training also contributes to improving the general state of health and the feeling of well-being in women over 50.

Better body awareness increases quality of life and daily well-being - those who are comfortable in their body gain more self-confidence and self-awareness. Training in particular for the back, arms and pectorals improves posture and is especially useful for preventing the negative consequences of sedentary work.

An advantage for women with little time and limited budget is that strength training can also be done at home, without necessarily having to join the gym. Using fitness equipment, such as kettlebells or dumbbells, it is possible to perform an effective workout even at home. It only takes half an hour to effectively train the whole body.

How long and how many times a week should you do strength training as a woman over 50?
The frequency of strength training depends on your starting point. For beginners, 2 training sessions per week is already enough, while if you are already experienced and well trained you can easily train the whole body 3 times a week. Make

sure you give your muscles enough time to recover and plan at least one rest day between workouts. Muscle growth occurs during the recovery phase. Therefore, in this case the fundamental rule of life applies: less is more.

When training strength, you don't need to spend hours in the gym. If you want to develop muscles, your training should not last more than 60-90 minutes. If you train for too long, the stress hormone, called cortisol, is released. This can lead to a lack of results and cause you to no longer see progress.

Also, don't forget to increase the difficulty of your exercises over time. You can do this, for example, by increasing the reps or by using a heavier weight. Important: a clean execution always remains the focus of your training!

Effective exercises for a dream body
Especially the fundamental exercises, in strength training for women, are very effective for training the synergy between the different muscle groups. This aspect is essential for a correct and healthy posture and for performing movements

well in daily life and in sport. It is no coincidence that these exercises have established themselves as true classics.

The most important fundamental exercises are: weight lifting, squats, lunges, Bench Press, pull-ups.

The unbeatable benefits of the fundamental exercises are the following.
- they train multiple parts of the body at the same time;
- minor muscle groups are also involved and are often neglected in other exercises;
- thanks to complexity and effort, fat burning increases;
- they stimulate the production of the growth hormone testosterone which acts on the whole body;
- hardly any tools or objects are needed, the exercises can be performed at home and made more difficult through variations.

Example training program for women
At the beginning it is enough to train 2-3 times a week. It is possible to integrate an endurance training session. The training program can be configured, for example, as you can see on the next page.

Monday	Strength training A (Bench Press, Military Press, crunches)
Tuesday	Rest
Wednesday	Strength training B (weightlifting, pull-ups, rowing machine)
Thursday	Endurance session (30 minutes of cycling)
Friday	Strength training C (squats, lunges, leg press)
Saturday	Rest
Sunday	Endurance session (30 minutes of jogging)

It is important to include breaks in your training program, as this gives your body time to recover before the next session and build new muscle mass. This is particularly true if you are on an intermittent fasting regimen, where you are constantly in a caloric deficit.

To understand how to perform these exercises in the correct way, we advise you to ask your local gym instructor.

Chapter 8 - Practical Steps to Get Started with Intermittent Fasting

In the previous chapters we have laid out the foundations for what is coming in the next pages. In fact, if you have gone through the previous chapters, by now you should have a clear idea on what intermittent fasting is, how it works and have some basic concepts of nutrition.

In this chapter we get on the bread and butter of this book. In fact, we will tell you how to practically start an intermittent fasting plan.

Intermittent fasting involves an overall change in diet and lifestyle, because instead of reducing calorie intake or eliminating certain food groups, it regulates the hours during which you can eat. Typically, fasting also includes hours of sleep and prohibits eating until it ends. There are several ways to implement the intermittent fasting diet. Furthermore, it is possible to combine it with physical exercise and/or the reduction of calories in order to alleviate the inflammatory processes at a systemic level, but it is also able to lose weight and increase muscle mass.

Let's see the practical steps to start an intermittent fasting program.

Consult your doctor before starting
Talk to your doctor and explain that you are considering intermittent fasting. Ask about the positives and negatives of this diet, and be sure to let him know about any health problems you may be suffering from.
Intermittent fasting can have a significant effect on your daily metabolism. Do not fast without consulting your doctor in case of pregnancy or major medical conditions.
Warning: due to the intermittent frequency of food intake, type 1 diabetics following this dietary regimen may have difficulty regulating and maintaining normal insulin levels.

Choose time frames that you can stick to
When following this diet, you fast at certain times of the day (typically 16-20 hours a day) or even for 23 hours before making a full meal for the remaining 1, 4, or 8 hours. Intermittent fasting not only allows you to lose weight, but is also a great way to regulate and plan your food intake. It is important to establish and respect the times of daily fasting.

For example, you can gradually adopt this regimen by having only two meals a day. Choose a time to have your last meal of the day and stick to it.

Choose and respect the schedule

You must opt for times that allow you to take in about 2000 calories in the space of 24 hours if you are a man or 1500 if you are a woman. Rarely (or occasionally) you can indulge in snacks of 20-30 calories maximum until the end of the fasting window (a few sticks of carrot / celery or a quarter of an apple, 3 cherries, grapes / raisins, 2 small crackers or 30g of chicken / fish or something similar). In general, the times of intermittent fasting are essentially the same, they differ only by a few hours. You can choose between several methods. Some of the most popular ones are the following.

- **One meal window**. You fast for 23 hours a day and choose an interval of 1 hour a day (for example, 6:00 pm to 7:00 pm) to prepare your meals and eat healthy dishes.
- **Two meals Window**. You indulge in two healthy meals a day, one at 12pm and the other at 7pm. Then you fast for 17 hours after the second meal, sleep and don't eat breakfast until the fasting period is over.

- **Alternate days.** You fast on Mondays and Thursdays, but eat right on the other 5 days. Thus, the last meal could fall on Sunday evening, for example at 8pm. This method is called the "5: 2 diet" and allows you to eat 5 days and fast for the remaining 2 days.

Moderately decrease your daily calorie intake

If you typically consume 2000-3000 calories per day, you can reduce this amount slightly during the shorter intervals when you can eat. Try not to exceed 1500-2000 calories per day. To achieve this, customize your diet by including healthy carbohydrates, avoiding white bread and pasta, but incorporating complex carbohydrates and certain types of fats.

You will need to take in all your daily calories during one or two time windows when you are allowed to eat.

You may find that it's not that hard to cut down on calories because you won't have much time to consume them during the week.

Don't drastically change your diet

When you adopt intermittent fasting, you don't have to eliminate any particular food group (such as fat or carbohydrates). As long as you follow a healthy and balanced diet and don't exceed 2000 calories per day you can feed yourself as you always did before starting. Intermittent fasting changes the timing of food consumption, not the choice of dishes to eat.

However, if you find yourself consuming too many processed foods, we advise you to seek medical help from someone that is qualified to prescribe you a nutritional plan. Having healthy eating habits in the first place is the first step to a successful intermittent fasting diet.

A balanced diet includes only small amounts of processed foods, which are rich in sodium and added sugars. Opt for healthy proteins (from meat, including chicken and fish), fruits and vegetables, and moderate daily amounts of carbohydrates.

Gradually adopt the intermittent fasting diet

If you are not used to fasting, this regimen can affect your appetite, hunger and body functioning. You can adopt it little by little by extending the hours of fasting between meals or by starting not to eat one day a week. It will be beneficial to your body as it will allow it to detoxify and relieve unwanted symptoms (including headaches, low blood pressure, fatigue and irritability).

You can also indulge in some light snacks at first during fasting periods. A 100-calorie snack of proteins and fats (nuts, cheese, or protein bars) will not affect the effectiveness of the fast, neither at the start nor at the end. So, eat something very light.

In the meantime, gradually change your diet by reducing your consumption of processed foods, such as sausages, dairy products, and sodas.

Have the last meal before fasting

During the last meal before fasting, don't give in to the temptation to gorge yourself on junk food, sugars, and processed foods. Opt for fresh fruits and vegetables and get plenty of protein so you don't lower your energy levels. For example, you might consider chicken breast, a piece of garlic bread, and a salad made of lettuce, tomato, sliced onion, topped with vinaigrette.

Some people binge at first, although this behavior complicates digestion and impairs adaptation to the fasting phase in the period of food abstinence.

Eat a full meal before starting the fast. If you only consume foods rich in sugar or carbohydrates, you will be hungry again in a short time.

Load up on protein and fat when you can eat. It is not easy to maintain a low intake of carbohydrates and lipids because the sense of satiety is not satisfied and one always feels hungry during the fasting period.

Refrain from food when you sleep

That way you won't think about your stomach rumbling during a long fast. Get at least 8 hours of sleep each night and fast for at least a few hours before and after. When you wake up you will no longer be hungry because you know that you will soon be able to indulge in a big meal.

The first or main meal after fasting is the reward for being able to abstain from food. You'll be hungry, so indulge in a full meal.

Stay hydrated

Although you have chosen to fast during the day, this does not mean that you need to stop drinking. Indeed, it is essential to stay hydrated during your abstinence from food, so that the body continues to function properly. Opt for water, herbal teas, and non-calorie drinks.

By drinking you will also avoid feeling hunger pangs because liquids fill the stomach.

Set a goal for weight loss

The intermittent fasting diet can actually help you lose weight by decreasing your daily calorie intake and allowing your body to burn fat stores. By reducing the time you spend eating, you can shed excess body fat and speed up your metabolism. With intermittent fasting you will also be able to alleviate systemic inflammatory processes.

If you are fasting because you are motivated by the desire to achieve a personal goal, you will have more mental strength to continue when things get difficult.

Increase lean muscle mass while fasting

This diet offers you an excellent opportunity to build muscle. Work out just before your first meal (or, if you eat twice a day, do it between meals). Your body will be able to use calories more effectively, so try to consume about 60% of your daily calories immediately after training. To stay healthy and gain muscle mass, don't cut your calorie intake to less than 10 calories per 500g of body weight.

For example, a 60kg woman should consume at least 1200 calories per day to lose weight without starving, by combining this regimen with moderate training. If you eliminate an excessive amount of calories you risk getting sick and not toning the muscle structure.

Customize your workout so you have the physique you want

The sport to choose during the intermittent fasting diet depends on the results you want to achieve. If you're simply trying to lose weight, focus on aerobic activity and cardiovascular exercise (like the ones described in the dedicated chapter). If you want to gain and tone muscle mass, you will need to opt for anaerobic training, such as weight lifting. Again, refer to the previous chapters for a detailed training plan.

If you want to lose weight, do aerobic or cardiovascular exercise in long sessions.

If you want a more muscular body, opt for anaerobic activity, characterized by intense but short-term efforts, which do not suddenly accelerate the heart rate. As we have already seen, this type of training is based on resistance exercises or weight lifting, not on long sessions of aerobic or cardiovascular activities.

Chapter 9 - Before Fasting

If in the previous chapter we have talked about the basic strategies to start fasting, now we have to point out some key concepts to follow in order to start your intermittent fasting diet with ease.

By following these ideas, you make sure to stay healthy and safe from the start. Once again, if you have questions, doubts or are not sure on how to approach this diet, follow the advice of your doctor.

Fasting means stopping food and drink for a specific period. People choose to fast to cleanse their digestive system, to lose weight, and in some cases, for spiritual or religious reasons.

Consult your doctor well in advance
During the fasting period, taking certain medications could be dangerous and have adverse effects on your health due to changes in blood chemistry. Fasting may not be suitable for people with particular health conditions, such as pregnancy, advanced cancer, low blood pressure, etc. Furthermore, your

doctor will likely give you a urine or blood test before the fast begins.

Determine the type and duration of fasting you want to practice

Among the numerous ways of fasting we find water fasting, juice fasting, spiritual fasting, slimming fasting, etc. As we have seen, fasting can be extended from 1 to 30 days, depending on your specific goal. Research different fasting practices and choose the one that best suits your health condition and needs.

Be prepared for the changes that will take place in your body

As a result of the detoxification process, fasting can cause side effects such as diarrhea, exhaustion, fatigue, weakness, increased body odor, headache and more.

Consider taking a vacation from work or taking some time to relax throughout the day to limit the effects of fasting on your body.

It is important to know in advance the possible side effects caused by fasting, make sure that your research and your information are correct, detailed and comprehensive.

1 to 2 weeks before you start your fast, reduce your normal intake of addictive substances and break your eating habits. This procedure will reduce the potential withdrawal symptoms that you may experience during the fasting period. Addictive substances include alcohol, caffeinated beverages (such as tea, coffee, and carbonated drinks), cigarettes, and cigars.

Change your diet 1 to 2 weeks in advance
This means following these simple advice.
- Reduce your intake of chocolate and other foods that contain refined sugars and high percentages of fat.
- Reduce portion sizes during meals.
- Reduce the amount of meat and dairy you eat.
- Increase your intake of raw or cooked vegetables and fruit.
- In the days immediately before the fast begins, limit the amount of food you eat.
- Eat only raw fruits and vegetables, they will help cleanse and detox your body by preparing it for the fasting period.
- Drink only water and fresh, freshly prepared fruit and vegetable juices.

And most importantly, do not overthink what you are doing. We have stressed out how important it is to do things the right way, but we want to emphasize the fact that overthinking the process will not yield greater results. Just stay calm and collected during the entire process and you will start burning fat like crazy.

Chapter 10 - After Fasting

As we have stated from the start, intermittent fasting is a type of diet that cannot be conducted for extremely long periods of time due to the fact that it is highly stressful for the body and the mind. Especially for women of your age, we recommend not to exaggerate and limit this diet to 2 week cycles.

Once you have finished a cycle, we recommend you follow these tips to get back to your normal eating habits.

When breaking an intermittent fasting cycle, it is important to act with caution to make it easier for the body to restore a normal digestive process. Since your digestive system will most likely have reduced enzyme production and affected stomach mucus, eating too much or ingesting certain foods too quickly could cause malaise, including nausea, stomach pain, or dysentery. Returning to a normal meal slowly and strategically will help you break your fast safely, without causing any disruption to your digestive system.

Set a deadline based on the length of your intermittent fasting cycle

It is important to know the time frame in which to stop it. Normally, the length of the fast will determine the length of time needed to break it. Do not neglect the initial stages of the interruption, otherwise you will ruin all the work done and you will stop feeling good.

For longer intermittent fasting cycles you will need to provide a break time of 4 days. The first two days you will have to limit yourself to a very slight reintroduction of basic foods, and then start adding more.

For shorter intermittent fasting cycles give your body 1 to 3 days of recovery. On the first day, you will only be able to take fruit juices and perhaps some broth. Depending on your state of well-being, you will be able to take faster steps over the next two days.

For a 1 day intermittent fasting cycle, dedicate 1 or 2 days to your recovery. Your system may not have been placed under high stress, but you won't be able to immediately resume eating the wrong foods.

Plan your meals

Creating a specific meal plan, for the length of time it takes to reintroduce food into your system, will help you avoid making mistakes by consuming food you should avoid to keep weight off. An example of food planning (to break a four-day intermittent fasting cycle) would be the following.

- Day One. Two 240ml cups of fruit / vegetable juice (carrots, green leafy vegetables, banana, apple) diluted 50% with water 4 hours apart.
- Day Two. Plus diluted fruit / vegetable juice with bone broth and 110 grams of fruit (pears and watermelon) every 2 hours.
- Day Three. 240 ml of yogurt and fruit juice for breakfast, snack with 110 grams of watermelon and vegetable juice, lunch with vegetable soup and fruit juice, snack with 110 grams of apple, for dinner leafy vegetables topped with yogurt and fruit juice.
- Day Four. Soft-boiled egg with fruit juice for breakfast, yogurt and berries as a snack, beans and vegetables for lunch, apple and dried fruit for a snack, vegetable soup and fruit juice for dinner.

On day one, focus mostly on eating high quality fruit and vegetable juices. To start breaking fast, especially after a long intermittent fasting cycle, you need to rehydrate your body. To do this, on the first day or two, you will only need to drink diluted fruit and vegetable juices.

To break the fast, drink 240ml of diluted fruit or vegetable juice. Avoid those products that contain added sugars and additives. In fact, you just got rid of it by fasting.

Integrate fruit and vegetable juice with vegetable or bone broth. Depending on your body's well-being conditions, after another 4 hours, you can start adding broth to your diet. In order not to overload your system, it is good to give the body an adequate amount of time between one food and another. Without the right temporal precautions, processing and digesting food would be difficult, even if it is a simple broth.

Start introducing raw fruit into your diet, especially for short fasts. If your intermittent fasting cycle has been prolonged for two weeks or more, it is probably advisable to stick to a juice and broth regimen for a longer period of time. In the other cases, the time has come to move on to solid fruit. Many fruits are rich in water and easily digestible, and at the same time loaded with nutrients and energy. Your system needs foods that are easy to assimilate, which reactivate the digestive system without straining it.

At the end of the first day or the beginning of the second, you can decide to start introducing small amounts of fruit.
Among the most recommended and tolerated fruits: melons, watermelons, grapes, apples and pears.

During this time, avoid acidic fruits, such as lemons and oranges, and fibrous ones, such as pineapple. Fibrous fruits are more difficult to digest, while highly acidic ones can cause discomfort.

Include yogurt
It is a highly recommended food for breaking an intermittent fasting cycle. Yogurt will help repopulate the digestive tract with beneficial bacteria and enzymes removed by the intermittent fasting cycle. Such probiotics will facilitate the digestive process.

Introduce it during the second day, or when you start consuming fruits again. It is advisable to reintroduce the enzymes into the system as soon as possible, without overloading it.

Use only sugar-free yogurt, as sugar (in the processed variety and not the natural one contained in fruit) will negatively affect your health.

During this time, listen to your body
It will tell you if you are moving too fast. Some symptoms are normal, such as intense hunger or lightheadedness, as you haven't eaten consistently for a long time. In case of constipation, stomach cramps or vomiting (even just the

relative sensation) it will be good to go back to taking only diluted juices and broth.

Also pay attention to the foods that you are reintroducing into your diet, in fact you may find that you suffer from some food allergy. Notice how foods make you feel: nauseated, numb, itchy or heavy in your mouth or tongue.

Introduce the vegetables again
Start with leafy greens, such as lettuce and spinach. Eat them raw and use yogurt to make the dressing. Keep eating fruit and drinking juices as your body regulates its digestive system.

After eating lettuce and spinach, add more vegetables. Eat them both raw and cooked. If you wish, you can make a vegetable soup.

Sprouts are also a great choice, as they contain numerous minerals and antioxidants that are easy to digest and necessary for the body.

Add some grains and beans. You will need to cook them well and eat them in addition to fruits and vegetables. Your appetite will grow as you reintroduce different foods into your diet.

Try nuts and eggs after getting used to solid foods. The simplest way to eat eggs is to cook them soft-boiled or beaten. Hard-boiled eggs are more difficult for the body to digest.

Make sure your body feels good before introducing multiple foods. If you digest vegetables and fruit without difficulty (for example cramps, nausea, etc.), you can decide to eat more complex foods to process. But if you have had episodes of malaise up until now, wait before moving on. Trust in those foods that your body has gratefully enjoyed.

Eat small portions
After you complete your juice intake within 4 hours of each other, you will want to start by eating every two hours or so. Your body will gradually adapt to food, and you will make progress towards larger meals.
In the end, the ideal daily meal plan consists of 3 meals and 2 snacks. Once you have reached this milestone, your body will return to normal and, possibly, will feel better thanks to the successful purification.

Chew well
Chewing food breaks it down making it easier to digest. Therefore eat slowly and allow your body to prepare for digestion. Aim to chew each bite at least 20 times before

moving on to the next. This is a great idea even during your intermittent fasting cycle.

Understand that dysentery and frequent bowel movements are common symptoms following the regular reintroduction of solid foods after longer intermittent fasting cycles. On the first day, you will stick to watermelon juice and introduce grapes and pears into the second. Immediately after consuming only small portions of grapes and pears, you will experience episodes of dysentery, as solid foods will pass through your system.

Those who do intermittent fasting often experience these symptoms after reintroducing solid foods into their bodies on a regular basis. During the fast, the digestive system remained at rest and inactive. The intestinal enzymes have become unaccustomed to work. Suddenly, they are given solid food and have to reactivate in a very short time. Don't be surprised that they go wrong.

The solution is to stay on the track. In all likelihood, it's not the food that's the problem, it's the simple fact that you're asking your body to do something it's not ready for after an intermittent fasting cycle. Stick to mostly fruit and vegetable juices, accompanied by broths, and ingest something simple and solid only occasionally. Your body will readjust in a day or two.

Understand that flatulence and constipation are also common symptoms

If, unlike the case seen above, you will not be able to evacuate after reintroducing solid foods into your diet on a regular basis, do not be frightened. You are not a rare case, and you are not making any mistakes. Here's what you can do.

- Mix 1 teaspoon of Metamucil (or another fiber food supplement) and 1 teaspoon of aloe juice in 240 ml of water and drink the solution obtained before meals. The fiber supplement and aloe vera are both mild laxatives, which are supposed to promote a bowel movement.
- Avoid foods and drinks that cause or worsen constipation. Dried fruit, cabbage and coffee, while otherwise beneficial, could make your constipation worse in this case. Limit yourself to those fruits and vegetables that are easy to digest, such as plums, sweet potatoes, and squash.

Understand that too much variety, especially when reintroducing solid foods, can cause digestive problems. The key to effectively breaking an intermittent fasting cycle is simplicity. You can simply find a juice that suits your body and take nothing else for a day. The next day, find a simple, well-tolerated fruit and eat nothing else. Too many take it for granted that their digestive system is very resistant and punish it by giving it what they deem necessary, when in reality it is simplicity that it asks for. Choose the easy way out, your body will thank you.

During the first week, beware of oil-rich foods. Even foods that contain beneficial oils, such as nuts and avocados, can cause trouble for those stomachs that have only recently gotten used to solid foods again. Initially prefer fruits and vegetables without a large oil content, then notice your body's reactions to foods that are rich in them when you feel ready to reintroduce them.

If you follow these tips, we are sure you will have no problems reintroducing a standard diet after an intermittent fasting cycle.

Conclusion

We would like to thank you for making it to the end of this book. We have done our best to ensure that every information contained is useful and helps you in your weight loss journey.

We know how frustrating it could be to start an intermittent fasting protocol and feeling discouraged by the fact that results do not appear immediately. As we repeated throughout the book, the goal of intermittent fasting is to create a healthy lifestyle that can support you over the years, not just give you a rapid decrease in weight.

By following the tips shared in this book, you will certainly burn fat, lose weight and feel much better. However, as we do not know you in person, our final recommendation can only be the following one.

Before starting an intermittent fasting protocol talk to your doctor and find out whether intermittent fasting could be a good idea for you or not. Remember, never sacrifice your health to fit into that new skirt you just got.

Be healthy and your weight will adapt.

To your success!

Nancy Johnson

Lightning Source UK Ltd.
Milton Keynes UK
UKHW020647300421
382892UK00001B/77